Food Allergy

Editor

J. ANDREW BIRD

IMMUNOLOGY AND ALLERGY CLINICS OF NORTH AMERICA

www.immunology.theclinics.com

Consulting Editor
STEPHEN A. TILLES

February 2018 • Volume 38 • Number 1

ELSEVIER

1600 John F. Kennedy Boulevard • Suite 1800 • Philadelphia, Pennsylvania, 19103-2899

http://www.theclinics.com

IMMUNOLOGY AND ALLERGY CLINICS OF NORTH AMERICA Volume 38, Number 1

February 2018 ISSN 0889-8561, ISBN-13: 978-0-323-56984-2

Editor: Jessica McCool

Developmental Editor: Kristen Helm

Immunology and Allergy Clinics of North America (ISSN 0889–8561) is published quarterly by Elsevier Inc., 360 Park Avenue South, New York, NY 10010-1710. Months of issue are February, May, August, and November. Periodicals postage paid at New York, NY and additional mailing offices. Subscription prices are $333.00 per year for US individuals, $565.00 per year for US institutions, $100.00 per year for US students and residents, $411.00 per year for Canadian individuals, $220.00 per year for Canadian students, $717.00 per year for Canadian institutions, $445.00 per year for international individuals, $717.00 per year for international institutions, $220.00 per year for international students. To receive student/resident rate, orders must be accompanied by name of affiliated institution, date of term, and the *signature* of program/residency coordinator on institution letterhead. Orders will be billed at individual rate until proof of status is received. Foreign air speed delivery is included in all *Clinics* subscription prices. All prices are subject to change without notice. **POSTMASTER**: Send address changes to *Immunology and Allergy Clinics of North America,* Elsevier Health Sciences Division, Subscription Customer Service, 3251 Riverport Lane, Maryland Heights, MO 63043. **Customer Service: 1-800-654-2452 (U.S. and Canada); 314-447-8871 (outside U.S. and Canada). Fax: 314-447-8029. E-mail: journalscustomerservice-usa@elsevier.com (for print support); journalsonlinesupport-usa@elsevier.com (for online support).**

Reprints. For copies of 100 or more, of articles in this publication, please contact the Commercial Reprints Department, Elsevier Inc., 360 Park Avenue South, New York, New York 10010-1710. Tel. 212-633-3874, Fax: 212-633-3820, E-mail: reprints@elsevier.com.

Immunology and Allergy Clinics of North America is covered in MEDLINE/PubMed (Index Medicus), Current Contents/Life Sciences, Science Citation Index, ISI/BIOMED, Chemical Abstracts, and EMBASE/Excerpta Medica.

Contributors

CONSULTING EDITOR

STEPHEN A. TILLES, MD
Executive Director, ASTHMA Inc. Clinical Research Center; Partner, Northwest Asthma and Allergy Center; Clinical Professor of Medicine, University of Washington, Seattle, Washington, USA

EDITOR

J. ANDREW BIRD, MD
Associate Professor, Departments of Pediatrics and Internal Medicine, Division of Allergy and Immunology, The University of Texas Southwestern Medical Center, Dallas, Texas, USA

AUTHORS

KATRINA J. ALLEN, MBBS, FRACP, FAAAI, PhD
Professor, Centre of Food and Allergy Research, Murdoch Children's Research Institute, Department of Paediatrics, The University of Melbourne, Departments of Allergy and Clinical Immunology, and Gastroenterology and Clinical Nutrition, The Royal Children's Hospital, Melbourne, Victoria, Australia; Institute of Inflammation and Repair, The University of Manchester, Manchester, United Kingdom

THERESA A. BINGEMANN, MD
Allergy, Immunology and Rheumatology, Rochester Regional Health, Division of Pediatric Allergy and Immunology, University of Rochester School of Medicine & Dentistry, Rochester, New York, USA

J. ANDREW BIRD, MD
Associate Professor, Departments of Pediatrics and Internal Medicine, Division of Allergy and Immunology, The University of Texas Southwestern Medical Center, Dallas, Texas, USA

AMANDA COX, MD
Assistant Professor of Pediatrics, Icahn School of Medicine at Mount Sinai, Elliot and Roslyn Jaffe Food Allergy Institute, New York, New York, USA

CARLA M. DAVIS, MD
Associate Professor of Pediatrics, Section of Immunology, Allergy and Rheumatology, Baylor College of Medicine, Texas Children's Hospital, Houston, Texas, USA

JOAN H. DUNLOP, MD
Fellow, Division of Pediatric Allergy and Immunology, The Johns Hopkins University School of Medicine, The Johns Hopkins Hospital, Baltimore, Maryland, USA

MALIKA GUPTA, MD
Assistant Professor, Division of Allergy and Immunology, Department of Internal
Medicine, University of Michigan, Ann Arbor, Michigan, USA

CATHERINE HAMMOND, MD
Department of Pediatrics, The University of Tennessee Health Science Center, Memphis,
Tennessee, USA

KIRSI M. JÄRVINEN, MD, PhD
Division of Pediatric Allergy and Immunology, University of Rochester School of Medicine
& Dentistry, Rochester, New York, USA

DAVID JEONG, MD
Translational Research Program, Virginia Mason Medical Center, Seattle, Washington,
USA

CORINNE A. KEET, MD, PhD
Associate Professor, Division of Pediatric Allergy and Immunology, The Johns
Hopkins University School of Medicine, The Johns Hopkins Hospital, Baltimore,
Maryland, USA

JOHN M. KELSO, MD
Division of Allergy, Asthma and Immunology, Scripps Clinic, San Diego, California,
USA

EDWIN H. KIM, MD, MS
Assistant Professor of Medicine, Division of Rheumatology, Allergy and Immunology, The
University of North Carolina at Chapel Hill, Chapel Hill, North Carolina, USA

JENNIFER J. KOPLIN, PhD
Centre of Food and Allergy Research, Murdoch Children's Research Institute, The Royal
Children's Hospital, Melbourne, Victoria, Australia

BRUCE J. LANSER, MD
Assistant Professor, Department of Pediatrics, Division of Allergy and Clinical
Immunology, National Jewish Health, Denver, Colorado, USA; Assistant Professor,
Department of Pediatrics, University of Colorado School of Medicine, Aurora,
Colorado, USA

XIU-MIN LI, MD, MS
Professor, Department of Pediatrics, Division of Allergy and Immunology, Jaffe
Food Allergy Institute, Director, Center for Integrative Medicine for Immunology
and Wellness, Icahn School of Medicine at Mount Sinai, NY, USA

JAY A. LIEBERMAN, MD
Associate Professor, Department of Pediatrics, The University of Tennessee Health
Science Center, Memphis, Tennessee, USA

WENYIN LOH, MBBS, MRCPCH
Allergy and Immune Disorders, Murdoch Children's Research Institute, Melbourne,
Victoria, Australia; Allergy Service, Department of Paediatrics, KK Women's and
Children's Hospital, Singapore

EMILY C. McGOWAN, MD
Adjunct Assistant Professor of Medicine, Division of Allergy and Immunology, University of Virginia, Charlottesville, Virginia, USA; Division of Allergy and Clinical Immunology, Department of Medicine, The Johns Hopkins University School of Medicine, Baltimore, Maryland, USA

ANNA NOWAK-WĘGRZYN, MD, PhD
Associate Professor of Pediatrics, Icahn School of Medicine at Mount Sinai, Elliot and Roslyn Jaffe Food Allergy Institute, New York, New York, USA

CHRISTOPHER P. PARRISH, MD
Assistant Professor, Division of Allergy and Immunology, Department of Pediatrics, The University of Texas Southwestern Medical Center, Dallas, Texas, USA

RACHEL L. PETERS, PhD
Centre of Food and Allergy Research, Murdoch Children's Research Institute, Department of Paediatrics, The University of Melbourne, The Royal Children's Hospital, Melbourne, Victoria, Australia

MELISSA L. ROBINSON, DO
Fellow, Department of Pediatrics, Division of Allergy and Clinical Immunology, National Jewish Health, Denver, Colorado, USA; Fellow, Department of Pediatrics, University of Colorado School of Medicine, Aurora, Colorado, USA

PUJA SOOD, MD
Division of Pediatric Allergy and Immunology, University of Rochester School of Medicine & Dentistry, Rochester, New York, USA

MIMI TANG, MBBS, PhD
Allergy and Immune Disorders, Murdoch Children's Research Institute, Department of Paediatrics, The University of Melbourne, Allergy and Immunology, The Royal Children's Hospital, Melbourne, Victoria, Australia

ERIK WAMBRE, PhD
Translational Research Program, Benaroya Research Institute at Virginia Mason, Seattle, Washington, USA

JULIE WANG, MD
Associate Professor of Pediatrics, Icahn School of Medicine at Mount Sinai, Elliot and Roslyn Jaffe Food Allergy Institute, New York, New York, USA

JEFFREY M. WILSON, MD, PhD
Allergy and Immunology Fellow, Division of Allergy and Immunology, Department of Medicine, University of Virginia, Charlottesville, Virginia

Contents

This article summarizes the current state of play with regard to food allergy prevention. Food allergy prevention strategies focused on promoting timely introduction of allergenic foods (predominantly peanut) into the infant diet have recently been introduced in several countries. Additional prevention strategies currently under investigation include optimizing infant vitamin D levels, modulating the gut microbiota through use of probiotics, and preventing eczema to reduce the risk of food sensitization through a damaged skin barrier.

Understanding the epidemiology of food allergy is complicated by the difficulty of identifying it on a large scale. The prevalence of food allergy is higher in younger age groups and decreases with age. Allergy to peanut and egg seems to be more common in Northern Europe, the United States, Canada, and Australia compared with Southern Europe, Eastern Europe, and Asia, whereas shellfish and fish allergies may be more common in Asia. The rate of transient unrecognized food allergy may be high and variable recognition of food allergy may explain some of the differences seen in food allergy prevalence.

The gastrointestinal tract has an abundant mucosal immune system to develop and maintain oral tolerance. The oral route of administration takes advantage of the unique set of immune cells and pathways involved in the induction of oral tolerance. Food allergy results from a loss of oral tolerance toward ingested antigens. Oral immunotherapy is thought to initiate desensitization through interaction of an allergen with mucosal dendritic cells that initiate downstream immune system modulation through regulatory T cells and effector T cells.

Finding an effective curative treatment for food allergy is a research priority. Although oral immunotherapy (OIT) is effective at inducing desensitization, the temporary nature of this effect and high rates of adverse reactions have highlighted a need for novel strategies to improve tolerance induction and safety. One such strategy is the use of an adjuvant together with food immunotherapy to either suppress allergic reactions and/or modulate the underlying allergic immune response. In particular, the use of bacterial adjuvants seems to be a promising means of enhancing OIT-induced sustained unresponsiveness and warrants further investigation.

The prevalence of food allergy is increasing. Food allergy can be life threatening and there is no approved treatment available. Allergen avoidance and rescue medication remain the sole management tools. Complementary and alternative medicine (CAM) use is common in the United States; however, research into safety and efficacy for food allergy is limited. Continued scientific research into food allergy herbal formula 2, refined methods of formulation, purified compounds, and other modalities is needed. Traditional Chinese medicine is the main component of CAM in the United States. Conventional doctors, CAM practitioners, and patients' families must collaborate to comanage these patients.

Unlike traditional food allergies, immunoglobulin E is not a key mediator of eosinophilic esophagitis (EoE). Nonetheless, food antigens are important triggers of EoE, and allergists play an important role in management of this chronic disease. This article addresses insights into the diagnosis and management as it relates to our evolving understanding about the pathogenesis of EoE.

Food protein-induced enterocolitis syndrome (FPIES) is a non–immunoglobulin E–mediated food allergy that usually presents in infancy. Cow's milk, soy, and grains are the most common food triggers. FPIES can present as a medical emergency with symptoms including delayed persistent emesis or diarrhea that can lead to severe dehydration and hemodynamic instability with abnormal laboratory markers. Diagnosis often can be made based on clinical history and noted improvement in symptoms once the suspected triggers have been removed from the diet, with oral food challenge as the gold standard for confirmation of diagnosis in unclear cases.

The gold standard for diagnosis of immunoglobulin (Ig)E-mediated food allergy remains the oral food challenge, with serum IgE testing and skin-
prick testing serving as acceptable alternatives. However, the increase
in prevalence of food allergy (both physician diagnosed and patient suspected) has led patients to pursue a variety of other alternative diagnostic
procedures for suspected food allergy, which are reviewed in this article.
These procedures (IgG testing, electrodermal testing, cytotoxic testing,
provocation/neutralization, and applied kinesiology) have largely been unproven and may lead to unnecessary elimination diets.

IMMUNOLOGY AND ALLERGY CLINICS OF NORTH AMERICA

THE CLINICS ARE AVAILABLE ONLINE!
Access your subscription at:
www.theclinics.com

IMMUNOLOGY AND ALLERGY
CLINICS OF NORTH AMERICA

FORTHCOMING ISSUES

May 2018
The Airway and Exercise
J. Tod Olin and James H. Hull, Editors

August 2018
Mastocytosis
Mariana C. Castells, Editor

November 2018
Biomarkers in Allergy and Asthma
Flavia Hoyte and Rohit K. Katial, Editors

RECENT ISSUES

November 2017
Drug Hypersensitivity and Desensitization
Mariana C. Castells, Editor

August 2017
Angioedema
Marc A. Riedl, Editor

May 2017
Biologic Therapies of Immunologic Diseases
Bradley J. Chipps and Stephen P. Peters, Editors

ISSUE OF RELATED INTEREST

Pediatric Clinics of North America, February 2017 (Vol. 64, No. 1)
Undiagnosed and Rare Diseases in Children
Robert M. Kliegman and Brett J. Bordini, Editors
Available at: http://www.pediatric.theclinics.com/

THE CLINICS ARE AVAILABLE ONLINE!

Access your subscription at:
www.theclinics.com

Foreword

The Quest for Food Allergy Treatments: On Course and Gaining Steam...Finally

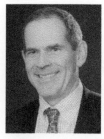

Stephen A. Tilles, MD
Consulting Editor

In the past decade, food allergy has become the largest unmet need among patients served by practicing allergists. This is due to a combination of a dramatic increase in the prevalence of food allergies, a lack of definitive therapy, and a reduction in unmet need for other common allergic diseases. Fortunately, appropriate forces have now mobilized to address the food allergy problem. This is analogous to an armada of military ships, including the "mother ship" of patients and doctors, together with "support ships" such as the NIH, FARE (Food Allergy Research and Education), physician specialty organizations such as the American College of Allergy, Asthma and Immunology and American Academy of Allergy, Asthma & Immunology, and the pharmaceutical industry. Thanks to the cooperation of these forces, and particularly the intensive translational and clinical research efforts that have been directed to food allergies, we now have a validated primary and secondary prevention strategy for peanut allergy; the first wave of FDA-approved immunotherapies is on the way, and a whole host of other treatment strategies, many involving biologics with novel immunological targets, are in early phases of development. This is great news for patients with food allergies. However, there are multiple levels of challenges to overcome in the short term, including educating primary physicians about appropriate primary prevention and helping practicing allergists with the logistics of overseeing oral immunotherapy and epicutaneous immunotherapy.

In this issue of *Immunology and Allergy Clinics of North America*, J. Andrew Bird, MD has impressively addressed each of these issues by engaging a group of well-respected authors to contribute articles that review topics ranging from currently accepted methods of prevention, diagnosis, and management, to emerging treatment strategies, and even complementary medicine approaches. The scope and timing of

Immunol Allergy Clin N Am 38 (2018) xiii–xiv
https://doi.org/10.1016/j.iac.2017.10.002
0889-8561/18/© 2017 Published by Elsevier Inc.

this issue qualify it as both a welcome addition to the literature and a practical reference for allergy specialists.

This is an exciting time for food allergy. After two decades of observing the epidemic grow without any new management options, we are entering a "golden age" during which we will partner with patients to discuss and provide new therapeutic options knowing that the armada is on course at full speed toward finding more definitive cures.

Stephen A. Tilles, MD
ASTHMA Inc. Clinical Research Center
Northwest Asthma and Allergy Center
University of Washington
9725 Third Avenue NE
Suite 500
Seattle, WA 98115, USA

E-mail address:
stilles@nwasthma.com

Preface

Food Allergy

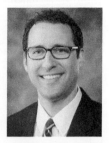

J. Andrew Bird, MD
Editor

Immunology and Allergy Clinics of North America last published an issue dedicated to the subject of food allergy following the release of the National Institute of Allergy and Infectious Diseases Guidelines for the Diagnosis and Management of Food Allergy in the United States in 2012. Since 2012, some aspects of our field remain unchanged. We continue to perceive a rising incidence of food allergy, an absence of an FDA-approved therapy for treatment of food allergy, and a growing recognition of other food-induced allergic diseases such as eosinophilic esophagitis and food protein–induced enterocolitis syndrome. However, there may be no 5-year period of more substantial progress in food allergy research than the period between 2012 and 2017.

Few studies have had the potential impact on disease prevention as what may be expected from dietary introduction recommendation changes as a result of the LEAP trial. NIH- and industry-funded trials investigating interventional therapeutics for treatment of life-threatening food allergies have accelerated, and we hope to have an FDA-approved product on the market within the next few years. An increasing amount of literature related to food allergy requires constant vigilance in order to appropriately counsel our patients and colleagues on the newest developments and possibilities for change in the near future.

The authors of this issue were chosen not only for their contributions toward the advancement of the study of food allergy but also for their reputations as astute clinicians who provide valuable examples to all of us as we care for patients with food-induced allergic diseases. It is my hope that these contributions will serve researchers and physicians as a valued resource in caring for and understanding our patients with food allergies. I want to especially thank the authors for their time in preparing excellent, current updates on the diagnosis, treatment, and latest advances in food allergy. Thank you to Dr Stephen Tilles for giving me the opportunity and freedom to develop this issue. A very special thanks is indebted to our patients and their families, who teach us every day and give us a reason to urgently find a cure. And last but certainly

Immunol Allergy Clin N Am 38 (2018) xv–xvi
https://doi.org/10.1016/j.iac.2017.10.001
0889-8561/18/© 2017 Published by Elsevier Inc.

immunology.theclinics.com

not least, thank you to my wife, Brenda, and son, Jake. Their encouragement, love, patience, and support keep me grounded, smiling, and confident in a bright future.

J. Andrew Bird, MD
Departments of Pediatrics and Internal Medicine
Division of Allergy and Immunology
The University of Texas Southwestern Medical Center
5323 Harry Hines Boulevard
Dallas, TX 75390-9063, USA

E-mail address:
Drew.Bird@UTSouthwestern.edu

Prevention of Food Allergies

Jennifer J. Koplin, PhD[a], Rachel L. Peters, PhD[a,b],
Katrina J. Allen, MBBS, FRACP, PhD[a,b,c,d,e,*]

KEYWORDS

- Food allergy • Prevention • Peanut allergy • Egg allergy • Eczema • Vitamin D
- Infant feeding • Probiotics

KEY POINTS

- There is now good evidence that timely introduction of peanut into the infant diet reduces the risk of peanut allergy in high-risk infants.
- There is also some evidence that timely introduction of egg might reduce the risk of egg allergy, whereas the role of timing of introduction of other allergenic foods has not yet been established.
- Additional food allergy prevention strategies currently under investigation include optimizing infant vitamin D levels, modulating the gut microbiota through use of probiotics, and preventing eczema to reduce the risk of food sensitization through a damaged skin barrier.

INTRODUCTION

A population-level approach to food allergy prevention moved one step closer in 2015 to 2016, with a successful trial of early peanut introduction for preventing peanut allergy. This widely lauded landmark study resulted in definitive changes to infant feeding guidelines around the world. As a result of this successful trial and subsequent development and dissemination of new infant feeding recommendations, there is a very real possibility that new generations of infants born in countries with high food

Disclosure Statement: K.J. Allen has received speaker's honorarium from Danone, Nutricia, Nestle, Alphapharm, and Aspen. J.J. Koplin and R.L. Peters have nothing to declare.
[a] Centre of Food and Allergy Research, Murdoch Children's Research Institute, Royal Children's Hospital, Flemington Road, Parkville, Melbourne, Victoria 3052, Australia; [b] Department of Paediatrics, University of Melbourne, Royal Children's Hospital, Melbourne, Victoria 3052, Australia; [c] Department of Allergy and Clinical Immunology, Royal Children's Hospital, Melbourne, Victoria 3052, Australia; [d] Department of Gastroenterology and Clinical Nutrition, Royal Children's Hospital, Melbourne, Victoria 3052, Australia; [e] Institute of Inflammation and Repair, University of Manchester, Oxford Road, Manchester M13 9PL, UK
* Corresponding author. Murdoch Children's Research Institute, Royal Children's Hospital, Flemington Road, Parkville, Melbourne, Victoria 3052, Australia.
E-mail address: katie.allen@rch.org.au

allergy prevalence, such as the United Kingdom, the United States, and Australia, will have less food allergy than the generation before. However, further targeted research is still required to bridge some important knowledge gaps. This research includes the following:

- Monitoring the impact on prevalence of changed guidelines
- Developing prevention strategies for foods other than peanut
- Developing strategies to prevent cases of peanut allergy that do not respond to earlier allergen introduction

In this review, the authors discuss the current state of food allergy prevention. They highlight topics of ongoing research as well as areas where prevention strategies may continue to evolve as new research findings emerge.

THE CURRENT BURDEN OF IMMUNOGLOBULIN E–MEDIATED FOOD ALLERGIES AROUND THE WORLD

Food allergy is estimated to affect around 5% to 10% of infants and young children in developed countries. Data show that the incidence of food-induced anaphylaxis increased between the 1990s and 2010, particularly in children,[1–3] although it remains unclear to what extent this is due to an increase in food allergy prevalence, an increase in severe reactions among allergic individuals, or an increased number of reactions in the same pool of allergic people. A recent acceleration in rates of adolescent anaphylaxis supports the concept of a cohort effect with children born in the early stages of the increase in food allergy prevalence in the early 2000s now reaching adolescence.[1]

There are increasing published reports on food allergy prevalence from around the world, which reveal emerging significant differences in the prevalence between countries, although the reasons for these differences are not yet established. The Europrevall birth cohort study was designed to compare food allergy prevalence between countries by using a standardized study protocol in multiple European centers. Around 12,000 infants from 9 countries were recruited into a series of birth cohorts in 2005 to 2010, with approximately 9000 infants followed up to 2 years of age. The prevalence of egg allergy was reported to range from 0.07% in Greece to more than 2% in Germany and the United Kingdom,[4] whereas cow's milk allergy ranged from 0% in Greece to 1.3% in Lithuania.[5] Outside of Europe, the HealthNuts study in Australia recruited 12-month-old infants around the same time as Europrevall (2007–2011). Of the 5300 participating infants, 3.0% were peanut allergic, 9.0% egg allergic, and 0.8% sesame allergic.[6]

Recently, there have been new publications reporting the prevalence of food allergy in infants in South Africa and China, both countries where food allergy was previously considered to be rare. The South African Food Sensitization and Food Allergy study (SAFFA) used a population-based sampling frame to recruit an unselected cohort of infants aged 12 to 36 months.[7] In an interim analysis of the first 544 participants, the prevalence of challenge-proven immunoglobulin E (IgE)-mediated allergy was 2.5% (95% confidence interval [CI] 1.2–3.9), with a 1.8% prevalence of allergy to egg, 1.2% to peanut, and 0.2% to cow's milk. A study in Chongqing, China recruited 497 infants from 9 districts of Chongqing attending the Children's Hospital of Chongqing Medical University for routine heath checks, with a participation rate of 96% (477 of 497). The prevalence of challenge-proven food allergy was 3.8% (95% CI 2.5–5.9), with a 2.5% prevalence of egg allergy and 1.3% to cow's milk. Only 2 infants (0.4%) were sensitized to peanut and 1 to fish and shrimp; there were no positive challenges to peanut, fish, or shrimp.[8]

These recent studies of challenge-confirmed food allergy have provided strong baseline prevalence data. These data are a vital first step to measuring changes in food allergy prevalence in the future. Importantly, these baseline data will allow us to measure the extent to which new interventions, including a shift toward earlier introduction of dietary peanut, alter the prevalence of food allergy.

PREVENTION OF FOOD ALLERGY THROUGH TIMELY INTRODUCTION OF ALLERGENIC FOODS

In the late 1990s, most expert guidelines for prevention of allergic disease internationally recommended delayed introduction of allergenic solids, such as egg and peanut, until after 2 to 4 years of age, based on theoretic concerns regarding immaturity of the infant immune system. Later studies suggested that this was not effective in reducing increasing rates of food allergy; by 2008 there was increasing interest in earlier introduction of allergenic solids in a bid to engage an allergen-specific immune response and oral tolerance earlier in infancy.[9]

In 2008, Du Toit and colleagues[10] also observed that the common practice of earlier peanut consumption in Israel seemed to be associated with very low rates of peanut allergy. Jewish children in Israel had very little peanut allergy compared with Jewish children in the United Kingdom; most infants in Israel started eating peanut in the first year of life, whereas most infants in the United Kingdom avoided peanut until after 1 year of age. To test the hypothesis that earlier introduction of peanut could prevent peanut allergy in high-risk children, the group then mounted an intervention trial (the Learning Early About Peanut allergy [LEAP] study) whereby children with severe eczema and/or egg allergy were randomly assigned to either start eating peanut from 4 to 11 months of age or completely avoid peanut until 5 years of age.[11] Infants were first screened for possible peanut allergy by skin prick testing, and 11% of the screened infants were excluded from the study because they were already likely to be peanut allergic at 4 to 11 months of age (skin prick test wheal size >4 mm). In the remaining group of 640 infants, those who had consumed peanut starting from 4 to 11 months of age had an 81% relative reduction in peanut allergy compared with those who had avoided peanut. This study provided the first evidence from a randomized trial that delayed introduction of peanut into the diet of high-risk infants increased the risk of peanut allergy.

The results of trials for early introduction of other foods have been less clear. In an egg allergy trial, giving high doses of egg powder at 4 to 6 months of age to high-risk children (with eczema) seemed to be associated with some reduction in egg allergy risk compared with egg avoidance until 8 months of age; however, the difference between groups did not reach statistical significance and 31% of infants in the early egg introduction group had a reaction when the egg powder was first given, suggesting that egg allergy was already present at this early age in a significant proportion of infants with eczema.[12] A large trial of multiple allergenic food introductions from 3 to 6 months of age, compared with standard introduction from 6 months of age, did not find a significant difference in food allergy risk between the two groups in the primary intention-to-treat analysis.[13] There are several possible explanations for this finding, including low compliance with the intervention protocol, because a per-protocol analysis showed a possible protective effect of earlier introduction of both egg and peanut in those who were compliant with the intervention. Other studies of earlier egg introduction have also mostly reported a nonsignificant reduction in egg allergy with earlier egg consumption.[14] A recent systematic review and meta-analysis combined data from all of these studies and reported a reduction in egg allergy with introduction at 4 to 6 months of age compared with later introduction (risk ratio [RR] 0.56; 95% CI 0.36–0.87, P = .009). The same meta-analysis showed a potentially greater reduction in peanut allergy with early introduction (RR 0.29; 95% CI 0.11–0.74), with early introduction defined as 4 to 11 months of age.[14]

HOW MUCH FOOD ALLERGY CAN WE PREVENT THROUGH TIMELY INTRODUCTION OF ALLERGENIC FOOD?

Despite the great success of the early peanut introduction trial, likely peanut allergy (defined as a skin prick test wheal size >4 mm) was already present in around 11% of high-risk infants screened at 4 to 11 months of age. These infants were excluded from the intervention; early introduction of peanut is not a feasible intervention strategy for this group, because most are likely to react on consumption of peanut. Similarly, egg allergy prevention trials found relatively high levels of egg allergy already present by 4 months of age. The authors recently modeled the potential reduction in peanut allergy that could be expected if the LEAP study protocol was implemented for peanut allergy prevention in the general population. Their models predicted that around 40% to 60% of peanut allergy might be preventable under optimal conditions.[15] Although this is a substantial reduction in peanut allergy, there remains a need to identify strategies for individuals who do not benefit from early introduction.

To achieve even this level of reduction in peanut allergy, several questions regarding the optimal prevention strategy will need to be answered. One aspect that remains unanswered by LEAP is how much allergen exposure is enough to prevent food allergy. The editorial article[16] accompanying the publication of the trial results suggests that infants include 2 g of peanut protein 3 times a week for at least 3 years based on the intervention protocol, but little is known about the impact of variations in dosage of allergen exposure. Secondly, LEAP does not yet provide sufficient information about the critical window of opportunity of timing because peanut introduction occurred during a wide window from 4 to 11 months. Analysis of peanut introduction by restricted time windows and the impact of this on the risk of peanut allergy will be valuable as will mechanistic studies assessing immunologic and epigenetic differences based on the age of recruitment. Finally, there is as yet no evidence as to whether early introduction of peanut is equally effective in infants without eczema or egg allergy in infancy, a population in which approximately one-quarter of all peanut allergy cases occur.[15]

PREVENTING FOOD ALLERGY THROUGH TIMELY INTRODUCTION OF ALLERGENIC FOODS: ARE ALL FOOD ALLERGIES THE SAME?

It is not clear that timely introduction of allergens into the diet will be equally effective for preventing all food allergies. There are differences in allergic responses to different food allergens, and differences in the natural history of food allergy, with individuals more likely to outgrow their milk and egg allergy early in life compared with peanut allergy.[17] There is also some evidence of a variation in risk factors for different food allergy phenotypes.[18] In addition, the usual timing and amount of allergen given in the infant diet differs for different foods, with foods such as tree nuts and shellfish, often not given until later in childhood. Observational studies also suggest potentially different windows of opportunity for optimal introduction of different foods, with cow's milk introduction potentially needing to be earlier than egg or peanut.[19,20] There may not be a one-size-fits-all approach to preventing all food allergy, and the definition of timely introduction may be allergen specific.

Tree nuts are some of the most common foods to cause IgE-mediated allergic reactions and account for around 18% to 40% of all fatal food reactions.[21] Despite this, there have been far fewer studies of tree nut allergy prevalence and risk factors compared with peanut allergy. The authors recently reported that tree nuts were the second most common cause of food allergy in the adolescent age group after peanut, affecting 2.3% of the population.[22] There have been no studies of tree nut allergy in infants or young children; thus, it is not known whether tree nut allergy, like peanut allergy, also develops during infancy and whether it shares similar risk factors to peanut allergy. To date there have also been no prevention trials for tree nut allergy, with existing research focusing on peanut, egg, and cow's milk allergies.

HOW RELEVANT IS EARLY PEANUT INTRODUCTION IN COUNTRIES WITH LOW PEANUT ALLERGY PREVALENCE?

In countries with a low prevalence of peanut allergy where peanut is already introduced early, such as Israel, changes are unlikely to be required because the current practice seems to be safe and effective. It is not clear what to recommend for countries with a low prevalence of peanut allergy and low peanut consumption in infancy, which seems to be the case in Singapore.[23] Other areas of Asia also report low rates of peanut allergy, although data on infant peanut consumption have not yet been reported.[8] Although changes to infant feeding practices in these countries currently seem unnecessary, it may be advisable to continue to monitor any changes in peanut allergy prevalence with increases in industrialization.

BARRIERS TO ACHIEVING OPTIMAL TIMING OF INTRODUCTION OF ALLERGENIC FOODS

In order for infant feeding guidelines to be effective in reducing the population prevalence of peanut allergy, these guidelines need to result in changes in behavior. It is not yet clear to what extent parents will follow new guidelines recommending earlier peanut introduction. This change is the second major change in recommendations around peanut introduction in the past 10 years. In the late 1990s and early 2000s, many guidelines recommended delaying introduction of peanut until 1 to 3 years of age.[9] This advice was removed from most of these guidelines around 2008. The authors previously documented an evolving significant shift toward earlier introduction of peanut and egg 1 year after the removal of advice to delay peanut introduction in 2008.[24] Overall, however, less than 10% of the population changed their practices between 2007 and 2011; there was no significant change in the group with a family history of allergy, who might benefit the most from early allergen introduction because of their increased food allergy risk.

There may now have been a larger shift toward earlier introduction of allergenic foods, because updated guidelines specifically recommend early introduction, including for those at high risk of food allergy, and because of widespread media reporting of the trial results showing early introduction of peanut is protective. However, it will be important to monitor both awareness and uptake of these recommendations to ensure high compliance with earlier peanut introduction, particularly among infants with eczema or egg allergy.

The issue of whether high-risk infants should undergo screening for peanut sensitization before the first introduction of peanut into the diet remains the subject of debate.[25] Currently, some countries, such as Australia, recommend early introduction of peanut for all infants without screening, in a setting where infants at highest risk (particularly those with other food allergies) are often already under the care of an allergist. By contrast, recommendations in the United States by the National Institute of Allergy and Infectious Disease are for evaluation with peanut-specific IgE and/or a skin prick test and, if necessary, an oral food challenge before peanut introduction for the highest-risk infants (those with severe eczema, egg allergy, or both). Arguments for screening center around reducing the risk of reactions on first peanut consumption and promoting early introduction in high-risk groups when parents may be less willing to introduce peanut because of a fear of an allergic reaction. Arguments against screening include the difficulty in accommodating screening demands within the existing allergy workforce and a potential detrimental delay in the introduction of peanut while parents await specialist evaluation for their infant. The relative efficacy of these different strategies for both promoting timely peanut introduction and preventing peanut allergy remains to be seen.

IS THERE A ROLE FOR OTHER PREVENTION STRATEGIES APART FROM TIMING OF INTRODUCTION OF ALLERGENIC FOODS?

Changing the age at which infants are exposed to individual allergenic foods, such as peanut, has been shown to have an allergen-specific protective effect for peanut allergy but is unlikely to have a broader protective effect for all food allergies. In addition, the infants shown to benefit from early peanut introduction for peanut allergy prevention already had other manifestations of allergic disease (eczema and egg allergy). Therefore, development of other strategies that modulate the immune system to more broadly protect against the development of allergic responses to all food allergens remains an important research focus. Strategies that are currently under investigation include optimizing infant vitamin D levels, use of probiotics, as well as eczema prevention.

Vitamin D

Both ecological and epidemiologic evidence suggest a role of vitamin D in the development of food allergy. Several studies have shown higher rates of food allergy, adrenaline-autoinjector prescriptions, and hospital admissions for food-related anaphylaxis in children living further from the equator and those born in winter/autumn compared with summer/spring, both proxies of low vitamin D levels.[26–32] Vitamin D is associated with immune functioning, and it has been shown to suppress the T-helper type 2 (Th2) response, which is associated with B-cell production of IgE antibodies and food allergy; however, the exact immunologic mechanisms driving the role of vitamin D in the development of food allergy have not been established.

Direct evidence assessing vitamin D levels in infants and the risk of food allergy has only recently become available. The HealthNuts study in Australia provided the first evidence that a directly measured vitamin D level is associated with the risk of food allergy; infants with vitamin D levels less than 50 nmol/L at 1 year of age had an increased risk of challenge-confirmed peanut allergy at 1 year of age by 11-fold (adjusted odds ratio [aOR] 11.51; 95% CI 2.01–65.79) and egg allergy nearly 4-fold (aOR 3.79; 95% CI 1.19–12.08).[33] However, a smaller (n = 274) case-control study also in Australia did not find an association between vitamin D insufficiency at birth or 6 months of age and food allergy at 1 year of age.[34] A cross-sectional study in New Zealand reported a 2-fold increased risk of parent-reported doctor-diagnosed food allergy in children aged 2 to 5 years with vitamin D levels greater than 75 nmol/L compared with those with vitamin D levels of 50 to 74 nmol/L, although measurement of vitamin D levels occurred after 2 years of age rather than in infancy when food allergy is likely to have developed.[35] There may be a U-shaped association, that is, an increased risk in individuals with both low and high levels of vitamin D, as has been suggested for high IgE levels.[36]

Well-designed randomized controlled trials (RCTs) are needed to assess the role of vitamin D supplementation as a preventative strategy for food allergy and to establish whether vitamin D has a causal role in the development of food allergy. Several studies assessing maternal and postnatal vitamin D supplementation have failed to demonstrate a protective benefit against respiratory and allergic outcomes in their offspring.[37–39] This lack of beneficial effect may be because maternal administration of vitamin D is not the optimal route to impact on child outcomes. To date, there are no completed RCTs assessing vitamin D supplementation in infancy to prevent food allergy. The VITALITY study, an RCT investigating the use of vitamin D supplementation in infancy to prevent food allergy, is currently underway.[40]

Probiotics

Observational studies have shown that factors associated with increased microbial exposure, such as exposure to pet dogs, living on a farm, childcare attendance, and the presence of older siblings, may have a protective effect against developing food allergy.[41,42] The role that microbial exposure may play in the development of food allergy is described by the hygiene hypothesis, which postulates that a lack of exposure to microbes and infections in early childhood increases susceptibility to allergic disease by modulating the development of the immune system.[43] The gut microbiota plays an important role in the development and healthy functioning of the immune system, and its role in the development of food allergy has been a subject of interest in the scientific community. Disruption of the gut microbiota in infancy when the immune system is developing alters the Th1/Th2 balance in the intestinal mucosa and may contribute to the development of Th2-dependent allergic disease.[44–46]

Probiotics are live microorganisms, such as bacteria belonging to the Lactobacillus and Bifidobacterium groups, and can modulate the immune response by stimulating production of Th1 cytokines, suppressing the Th2 allergic response. Therefore, probiotic supplementation is another plausible target for both the prevention and treatment of allergic disease. Studies assessing probiotic supplementation have tended to use food sensitization as an outcome rather than challenge-proven food allergy. In 2014, the World Allergy Organization conducted a systematic review and meta-analysis of RCTs assessing probiotic supplementation for allergy prevention. They found no evidence to support that probiotic supplementation reduced the risk of food allergy, although probiotic use in pregnancy, breastfeeding, and infancy reduced the risk of eczema in infants, with low-certainty evidence requiring caution in interpretation of these findings.[47,48] In 2016, another meta-analysis found that probiotic supplementation when administered both prenatally and postnatally reduced the risk of food sensitization (RR 0.77; 95% CI 0.61–0.98), although there was no protective effect demonstrated when probiotics were administered only prenatally (RR 1.01; 95% CI 0.66–1.55) or only postnatally (RR 1.43; 95% CI 0.94–2.18).[49] Further studies on the use of probiotics as a prevention strategy for food allergy using challenge-proven outcomes are needed.

Eczema Prevention

A history of eczema is one of the strongest known risk factors for food allergy. A recent population-based study of more than 5000 infants showed that those with eczema were approximately 5 times more likely to develop food allergy than infants without eczema. One in 5 infants with eczema had challenge-confirmed allergy to egg white, peanut, or sesame by 12 months of age, compared with only 1 in 25 infants without eczema.[50] The risk of food allergy increased with an earlier age at onset and increasing severity of eczema, with approximately 50% of infants whose eczema started in the first 3 months of life and required treatment with topical corticosteroids developing a food allergy.

Skin barrier dysfunction is a feature of eczema and is thought to play an important role in the initiation of allergic sensitization and subsequent progression to food allergy and other allergic disease.[51–53] Therefore, prevention of eczema in early life may have a follow-on effect of preventing food allergy and other allergic diseases later in childhood.

One of the primary targets for eczema prevention is improving skin barrier integrity through regular application of a moisturizing cream in infants. RCT evidence supports efficacy of this intervention for reducing eczema.[54,55] However, it is yet to be determined whether prevention of eczema in early life will subsequently prevent allergic sensitization and food allergy. In an RCT of 118 high-risk infants, moisturizer was applied daily for the first 32 weeks of life (n = 59) and reduced the incidence of eczema by 32%. However, this trial failed to show an effect of the intervention on reducing egg sensitization at 32 weeks of age. Sensitization to other food and inhalant allergens was not measured.[54] A recent pilot RCT (n = 80) of twice-daily application of a ceramide-dominant moisturizing cream for the first 6 months of life showed a trend toward reduced eczema in the intervention group at 12 months of age (RR 0.32; 95% CI 0.07–1.51), although this did not reach statistical significance. Per protocol analysis showed a significant reduction in food sensitization at 12 months of age in the intervention group (0% vs 19.4%, P = .04), although this was not significant on intention-to-treat analysis.[56] The results of this pilot study are promising; further larger trials are needed, incorporating challenge-proven food allergy outcomes, to assess the potential of eczema prevention as a preventive strategy for food allergy.

SUMMARY

New food allergy prevention strategies, focused on promoting timely introduction of allergenic foods (predominantly peanut) into the infant diet, have been introduced in several countries. Additional prevention strategies are currently under investigation and are likely to expand our knowledge for foods other than peanut and how to prevent cases that are not preventable through timely allergen introduction in the infant diet. It will be important to monitor population responses to, and effectiveness of, existing and new prevention strategies as they are implemented and to have mechanisms in place to allow rapid adaption of prevention guidelines if necessary as new data come to light.

REFERENCES

1. Mullins RJ, Dear KB, Tang ML. Time trends in Australian hospital anaphylaxis admissions in 1998-1999 to 2011-2012. J Allergy Clin Immunol 2015;136(2):367–75.
2. Rudders SA, Arias SA, Camargo CA Jr. Trends in hospitalizations for food-induced anaphylaxis in US children, 2000-2009. J Allergy Clin Immunol 2014;134(4):960–2.
3. Turner PJ, Gowland MH, Sharma V, et al. Increase in anaphylaxis-related hospitalizations but no increase in fatalities: an analysis of United Kingdom national anaphylaxis data, 1992-2012. J Allergy Clin Immunol 2015;135(4):956–63.
4. Xepapadaki P, Fiocchi A, Grabenhenrich L, et al. Incidence and natural history of hen's egg allergy in the first 2 years of life - the EuroPrevall birth cohort study. Allergy 2016;71(3):350–7.
5. Schoemaker AA, Sprikkelman AB, Grimshaw KE, et al. Incidence and natural history of challenge-proven cow's milk allergy in European children - EuroPrevall birth cohort. Allergy 2015;70(8):963–72.

6. Koplin JJ, Wake M, Dharmage SC, et al. Cohort profile of the HealthNuts study: population prevalence and environmental/genetic predictors of food allergy. Int J Epidemiol 2015;44(4):1161–71.

7. Basera W, Botha M, Gray CL, et al. The South African food sensitisation and food allergy population-based study of IgE-mediated food allergy: validity, safety, and acceptability. Ann Allergy Asthma Immunol 2015;115(2):113–9.

8. Chen J, Hu Y, Allen KJ, et al. The prevalence of food allergy in infants in Chongqing, China. Pediatr Allergy Immunol 2011;22(4):356–60.

9. Koplin JJ, Allen KJ. Optimal timing for solids introduction - why are the guidelines always changing? Clin Exp Allergy 2013;43(8):826–34.

10. Du Toit G, Katz Y, Sasieni P, et al. Early consumption of peanuts in infancy is associated with a low prevalence of peanut allergy. J Allergy Clin Immunol 2008; 122(5):984–91.

11. Du Toit G, Roberts G, Sayre PH, et al. Randomized trial of peanut consumption in infants at risk for peanut allergy. N Engl J Med 2015;372(9):803–13.

12. Palmer DJ, Metcalfe J, Makrides M, et al. Early regular egg exposure in infants with eczema: a randomized controlled trial. J Allergy Clin Immunol 2013;132(2): 387–92.

13. Perkin MR, Logan K, Tseng A, et al. Randomized trial of introduction of allergenic foods in breast-fed infants. N Engl J Med 2016;374(18):1733–43.

14. Ierodiakonou D, Garcia-Larsen V, Logan A, et al. Timing of allergenic food introduction to the infant diet and risk of allergic or autoimmune disease: a systematic review and meta-analysis. JAMA 2016;316(11):1181–92.

15. Koplin JJ, Peters RL, Dharmage SC, et al. Understanding the feasibility and implications of implementing early peanut introduction for prevention of peanut allergy. J Allergy Clin Immunol 2016;138(4):1131–41.

16. Gruchalla RS, Sampson HA. Preventing peanut allergy through early consumption–ready for prime time? N Engl J Med 2015;372(9):875–7.

17. Peters RL, Koplin JJ, Gurrin LC, et al. The prevalence of food allergy and other allergic diseases in early childhood in a population-based study: HealthNuts age 4-year follow-up. J Allergy Clin Immunol 2017;140(1):145–53.

18. Peters RL, Allen KJ, Dharmage SC, et al. Differential factors associated with challenge-proven food allergy phenotypes in a population cohort of infants: a latent class analysis. Clin Exp Allergy 2015;45(5):953–63.

19. Katz Y, Rajuan N, Goldberg MR, et al. Early exposure to cow's milk protein is protective against IgE-mediated cow's milk protein allergy. J Allergy Clin Immunol 2010;126(1):77–82.

20. Koplin JJ, Osborne NJ, Wake M, et al. Can early introduction of egg prevent egg allergy in infants? A population-based study. J Allergy Clin Immunol 2010;126(4): 807–13.

21. McWilliam V, Koplin J, Lodge C, et al. The prevalence of tree nut allergy: a systematic review. Curr Allergy Asthma Rep 2015;15(9):54.

22. Sasaki M, Koplin JJ, Dharmage SC, et al. Prevalence of clinic-defined food allergy in early adolescence: the SchoolNuts study. J Allergy Clin Immunol 2017. [Epub ahead of print].

23. Tham EH, Lee BW, Chan YH, et al. Low food allergy prevalence despite delayed introduction of allergenic foods-data from the GUSTO cohort. J Allergy Clin Immunol Pract 2017. [Epub ahead of print].

24. Tey D, Allen KJ, Peters RL, et al. Population response to change in infant feeding guidelines for allergy prevention. J Allergy Clin Immunol 2014;133(2):476–84.

25. Tang MLK, Koplin JJ, Sampson HA. Skin testing is necessary before early introduction of peanut for prevention of peanut allergy: pro-con debate. J Allergy Clin Immunol Pract 2017 [Epub ahead of print].
26. Camargo CA Jr, Clark S, Kaplan MS, et al. Regional differences in EpiPen prescriptions in the United States: the potential role of vitamin D. J Allergy Clin Immunol 2007;120(1):131–6.
27. Hoyos-Bachiloglu R, Morales PS, Cerda J, et al. Higher latitude and lower solar radiation influence on anaphylaxis in Chilean children. Pediatr Allergy Immunol 2014;25(4):338–43.
28. Mullins RJ, Camargo CA. Latitude, sunlight, vitamin D, and childhood food allergy/anaphylaxis. Curr Allergy Asthma Rep 2012;12(1):64–71.
29. Mullins RJ, Clark S, Camargo CA Jr. Regional variation in epinephrine autoinjector prescriptions in Australia: more evidence for the vitamin D-anaphylaxis hypothesis. Ann Allergy Asthma Immunol 2009;103(6):488–95.
30. Mullins RJ, Clark S, Katelaris C, et al. Season of birth and childhood food allergy in Australia. Pediatr Allergy Immunol 2011;22(6):583–9.
31. Oktaria V, Dharmage SC, Burgess JA, et al. Association between latitude and allergic diseases: a longitudinal study from childhood to middle-age. Ann Allergy Asthma Immunol 2013;110(2):80–5.
32. Vassallo MF, Banerji A, Rudders SA, et al. Season of birth and food allergy in children. Ann Allergy Asthma Immunol 2010;104(4):307–13.
33. Allen KJ, Koplin JJ, Ponsonby AL, et al. Vitamin D insufficiency is associated with challenge-proven food allergy in infants. J Allergy Clin Immunol 2013;131(4): 1109–16.
34. Molloy J, Koplin JJ, Allen KJ, et al. Vitamin D insufficiency in the first 6 months of infancy and challenge-proven IgE-mediated food allergy at 1 year of age: a case-cohort study. Allergy 2017;72(8):1222–31.
35. Cairncross C, Grant C, Stonehouse W, et al. The relationship between vitamin D status and allergic diseases in New Zealand preschool children. Nutrients 2016; 8(6).
36. Hypponen E, Berry DJ, Wjst M, et al. Serum 25-hydroxyvitamin D and IgE - a significant but nonlinear relationship. Allergy 2009;64(4):613–20.
37. Chawes BL, Bonnelykke K, Stokholm J, et al. Effect of vitamin D3 supplementation during pregnancy on risk of persistent wheeze in the offspring: a randomized clinical trial. JAMA 2016;315(4):353–61.
38. Goldring ST, Griffiths CJ, Martineau AR, et al. Prenatal vitamin d supplementation and child respiratory health: a randomised controlled trial. PLoS One 2013;8(6): e66627.
39. Litonjua AA, Carey VJ, Laranjo N, et al. Effect of prenatal supplementation with vitamin d on asthma or recurrent wheezing in offspring by age 3 years: the VDAART randomized clinical trial. JAMA 2016;315(4):362–70.
40. Allen KJ, Panjari M, Koplin JJ, et al. VITALITY trial: protocol for a randomised controlled trial to establish the role of postnatal vitamin D supplementation in infant immune health. BMJ Open 2015;5(12):e009377.
41. Marrs T, Bruce KD, Logan K, et al. Is there an association between microbial exposure and food allergy? A systematic review. Pediatr Allergy Immunol 2013; 24(4):311–20.
42. Koplin JJ, Dharmage SC, Ponsonby AL, et al. Environmental and demographic risk factors for egg allergy in a population-based study of infants. Allergy 2012; 67(11):1415–22.

43. Strachan DP. Hay fever, hygiene, and household size. BMJ 1989;299(6710): 1259–60.
44. Shreiner A, Huffnagle GB, Noverr MC. The "microflora hypothesis" of allergic disease. Adv Exp Med Biol 2008;635:113–34.
45. Aitoro R, Paparo L, Amoroso A, et al. Gut microbiota as a target for preventive and therapeutic intervention against food allergy. Nutrients 2017;9(7).
46. Tsabouri S, Priftis KN, Chaliasos N, et al. Modulation of gut microbiota downregulates the development of food allergy in infancy. Allergol Immunopathol (Madr) 2014;42(1):69–77.
47. Cuello-Garcia CA, Brozek JL, Fiocchi A, et al. Probiotics for the prevention of allergy: a systematic review and meta-analysis of randomized controlled trials. J Allergy Clin Immunol 2015;136(4):952–61.
48. Fiocchi A, Pawankar R, Cuello-Garcia C, et al. World Allergy Organization-McMaster University guidelines for allergic disease prevention (GLAD-P): probiotics. World Allergy Organ J 2015;8(1):4.
49. Zhang GQ, Hu HJ, Liu CY, et al. Probiotics for prevention of atopy and food hypersensitivity in early childhood: a PRISMA-compliant systematic review and meta-analysis of randomized controlled trials. Medicine 2016;95(8):e2562.
50. Martin PE, Eckert JK, Koplin JJ, et al. Which infants with eczema are at risk of food allergy? Results from a population-based cohort. Clin Exp Allergy 2015; 45(1):255–64.
51. Lack G. Epidemiologic risks for food allergy. J Allergy Clin Immunol 2008;121(6): 1331–6.
52. Spergel JM, Paller AS. Atopic dermatitis and the atopic march. J Allergy Clin Immunol 2003;112(6 Suppl):S118–27.
53. Czarnowicki T, Krueger JG, Guttman-Yassky E. Novel concepts of prevention and treatment of atopic dermatitis through barrier and immune manipulations with implications for the atopic march. J Allergy Clin Immunol 2017;139(6):1723–34.
54. Horimukai K, Morita K, Narita M, et al. Application of moisturizer to neonates prevents development of atopic dermatitis. J Allergy Clin Immunol 2014;134(4): 824–30.e6.
55. Simpson EL, Chalmers JR, Hanifin JM, et al. Emollient enhancement of the skin barrier from birth offers effective atopic dermatitis prevention. J Allergy Clin Immunol 2014;134(4):818–23.
56. Lowe AJ, Su JC, Allen KJ, et al. A randomised trial of a barrier lipid replacement strategy for the prevention of atopic dermatitis and allergic sensitisation: the PEBBLES pilot study. Br J Dermatol 2017. [Epub ahead of print].

Prevention of Food Allergies

Epidemiology of Food Allergy

Joan H. Dunlop, MD, Corinne A. Keet, MD, PhD*

KEYWORDS

- Food allergy • Epidemiology • Prevalence • Age • Population • Geography
- Ethnic groups

KEY POINTS

- It is difficult to measure food allergy prevalence accurately in population-wide studies.
- In the United States, the estimated rate of self-reported food allergy is between 4.8% and 8% among children, whereas in international studies it is generally lower.
- An important exception is in Australia, where a high rate of food allergy in infants suggests that there may be substantial food allergy that is transient and not recognized.
- The rate of food allergy seems to be increasing, but data about fatalities and sensitization conflict with the increase seen in self-report and in hospitalizations.
- More data are needed to understand these trends.

In recent decades, food allergy has seemed to increase at a dizzying rate, sparking a search for the environmental factors that may underlie this increase. Understanding how many people are affected by food allergy, which groups are most at risk, and how risk has changed over time, that is, the epidemiology of food allergy, can provide clues to both genetic and environmental causes of the disease. Herein we review the epidemiology of food allergy, focusing on immunoglobulin E (IgE)-mediated allergy. Our perspective is from the United States, but we review international data to understand how geography and genetics may influence the development of allergy. We discuss the challenges inherent in efforts to estimate rates of food allergy, and summarize the conflicting evidence about whether increasing reports of food allergy reflect true increases in disease.

CHALLENGES IN UNDERSTANDING THE EPIDEMIOLOGY OF FOOD ALLERGY
Study Design

Estimating the rate of food allergy in a population is challenging because measuring food allergy on a large scale is difficult. True food allergy is defined by a specific,

Disclosure Statement: The authors have no disclosures to report.
Division of Pediatric Allergy and Immunology, Johns Hopkins University School of Medicine, The Johns Hopkins Hospital, CMSC 1102, 600 North Wolfe Street, Baltimore, MD 21287, USA
* Corresponding author.
E-mail address: ckeet1@jhmi.edu

reproducible, immunologically mediated clinical response upon exposure to allergen. Only food challenge directly assesses the clinical response upon allergic exposure, but the inherent risk to patients of food challenge, combined with the fact that it is time and staff intensive, makes it untenable in general for large-scale studies of food allergy prevalence, with few exceptions.

Self-report or parental report is easiest to obtain in broad population surveys, but generally tends to overestimate prevalence, because many people mistake intolerances, such as lactose intolerance, or other conditions for food allergy. Typically, population-based surveys ask brief questions that do not distinguish between IgE-mediated allergy, non–IgE-mediated allergy and intolerance, and many positive responses are not corroborated with further investigation.[1,2]

Surveys that use more detailed questions, such as those done by Gupta and co-workers[3] or Sicherer and associates,[4] may reduce overreporting but, because these surveys typically have food allergy as the focus and are done by telephone or Internet, they may suffer more from selection bias. Selection bias arises from the tendency for those with food allergy to be more likely to participate in surveys about food allergy. Soller and colleagues[5] quantified this bias in a telephone survey in Canada, and found that those who did not complete a full survey were much less likely to report food allergy than those who did. They estimated that selective nonresponse could inflate prevalence rates by somewhere between 20% and 110%. Further complicating matters, both nonresponse and overreporting of food allergy may vary between groups and over time.[6]

Objective measures of sensitization, such as specific IgE levels or skin-prick tests, have also been used in some national surveys to estimate food allergy rates. However, like self-report, these tests suffer from poor specificity, making it difficult to extrapolate prevalence estimates from sensitization data. As an example, Liu and associates[7] attempted to apply positive predictive values for food-specific IgE cutoffs to the National Health and Nutrition Examination Survey (NHANES) 2005 to 2006, the only national survey in the United States to prospectively measure food-specific IgE. Although the estimate of food allergy prevalence that they calculated, 2.5%, was similar to or less than estimates derived from self-report, the methods they used to derive this estimate may not be robust. This finding is because the positive predictive value is a function of both the inherent qualities of the test and the prevalence of disease in the population studied. Positive predictive values generated from allergy clinics with high rates of food allergy will lead to overestimates of food allergy when used in the general population. In fact, in that same survey, most of those assigned to "high probability of food allergy" reported eating the same food, making food allergy very unlikely.[8] Combining objective measures such as skin prick test or IgE with detailed questions about food allergy history would markedly improve the accuracy of population-based estimates of food allergy, but such surveys have not been done on a population wide basis in the United States to date.

Use data, such as that on hospitalizations and outpatient visits provide another window into the prevalence. However, these data are severely limited by the historical lack of specific and commonly used codes for food allergy, the fact that much food allergy may not present for medical care, and differences in health care use related to access to care.

Finally, a few population-based studies throughout the world have used food challenge to confirm food allergy. Among those efforts is the EuroPREVALL project, which sought to establish patterns of food allergy across Europe by establishing birth cohorts in 8 European countries.[9] Suspected food allergy was evaluated clinically, including with oral food challenge. In Australia, the HealthNUTs study surveyed 1-year-old children at immunization clinics with universal skin prick testing to select food allergens, and offered food challenge to anyone with positive skin prick tests.[10] As discussed in the section on egg allergy elsewhere in this article, this study raised the interesting possibility that, in addition to conflating food intolerance and true food allergy, questionnaire surveys may also miss some true, but transient, food allergy that is elicited during food challenge.

The Spectrum of Food Allergy

Another factor that complicates our understanding of the prevalence and risk factors for food allergy is that there is a spectrum of conditions that can broadly be called food allergy, but may have very different clinical implications. In the sections on milk and egg allergy, we discuss how most people with milk or egg allergy are able to tolerate highly cooked forms of these foods, confusing population-wide assessment of disease. Perhaps more important is oral allergy syndrome (OAS, also called pollen–food allergy syndrome), a syndrome caused by cross-reactivity to pollen allergens, and typically limited to oral symptoms. The most commonly implicated foods are fruits, vegetables, and nuts, and symptoms usually start in the second decade of life or later. Because symptoms can be very mild, it is often not recognized, but can also be confused with systemic food allergy. The prevalence is estimated to be at least 8% in the United States and likely higher in Europe, but is highly dependent on both age and geographic location.[11] Surveys that depend on questionnaire or IgE sensitization may be poorly able to distinguish this type of allergy from systemic food allergy.

The Effect of Age on Food Allergy Estimates

Worldwide, the prevalence of food allergy is higher in younger age groups, and decreases with age. Studies of birth cohorts suggest that this pattern of younger patients having higher rates of food allergy does not represent population shifts in prevalence. Rather, patients within the same birth cohort have peak of food allergy in early preschool years and then demonstrate a lower prevalence thereafter. For example, a birth cohort on the Isle of Wight in the UK, where food allergy was confirmed by oral food challenge, demonstrated a prevalence of 4% at 1 year of age,[12] 5% to 6% at 3 years of age,[13] and 2.5% at 6 years of age.[14] Similar results were seen in a Danish birth cohort with food allergy prevalence of 3.6% at 18 months and 1.2% at 72 months.[15] This trend is not always noted in questionnaire data, perhaps because OAS becomes more common with age, or perhaps because adults may be more likely to confuse intolerances with true allergies.

BEST ESTIMATES OF THE PREVALENCE OF FOOD ALLERGIES
Current Data on the Prevalence of Food Allergy in the United States

To date, nationally representative studies of food allergy in the United States are limited to questionnaire surveys. Among children, the estimated rate of food allergy was 6.5% in NHANES 2007 to 2010,[15] when food allergy questions were included in the dietary behaviors survey, 5.7% in the 2015 National Health Interview Survey, which asked about food or digestive allergy in the past 12 months[16]; 4.8% in the 2007 National Survey on Children's Health,[17] which asked the same question; and 8% in an Internet survey by Gupta and colleagues[3] focused on food allergy.

There are far fewer data about food allergy in adults in the United States. From the NHANES 2007 to 2010 data, the estimated rate of food allergy among adults was 9.7%[8] and in a survey using a consumer panel conducted by the US Food and Drug Administration, the rate was 13% in 2010.[18]

Global Differences in Food Allergy Prevalence

As in the United States, most of the data about global food allergy rates are obtained by self-report, although there are concerted efforts by several large groups to conduct studies where food allergy is confirmed by oral food challenge. Whether obtained by self-report or confirmed by food challenge, rates of food allergy overall and to specific foods are quite variable, even within surveys, regions, and countries.

Prescott and colleagues[19] recently conducted a global survey of World Allergy Organization member countries to try to understand geographic differences in the prevalence of food allergy. Using a standardized data collection tool, they estimated the prevalence of food allergy in 89 countries spanning Europe, Asia/Oceania, the Americas, Africa, and the Middle East. Among infants and preschool aged children, the estimated rate of food allergy in data derived from questionnaire or questionnaire plus sensitization ranged from 2.5% to 5% in Sweden, France, Japan, and Taiwan to highs of almost 10% in Finland and Canada, with Hong Kong and Korea somewhere in between. Among children older than 5, the estimated prevalence varied more widely, from more than 10% or even 15% in Italy, Ghana, Colombia, Lithuania, Iceland, Tanzania, and Mozambique to less than 5% in Kenya, France, Estonia, Israel, and Australia. Among adults, the self-reported rate of doctor-diagnosed food allergy in the EuroPrevall community surveys was 4.4% overall, with country-specific estimates ranging from 0.5% in Lithuania to 7.8% in Switzerland.[20]

Far fewer studies have confirmed questionnaire report with food challenge. Among infants and preschoolers, rates of food allergy confirmed by oral food challenge range from a low of 1% in a city in Thailand,[21] to 3% in an urban area of China,[22] to a 5% cumulative incidence before the age of 2 in the UK,[23] to a high of 10% in Australia.[10] Among older children, prevalence ranges from 0.16% among adolescents in Turkey,[24] 1.2% among 6-year-old children in Denmark,[25] to 2.5% among 6-year-old children on the Isle of Wight in the UK.[26] Very few prevalence data were derived via oral food challenge for adults, but 1 Danish study found a prevalence of 3.2% in an unselected population.[27]

In sum, the global data are somewhat confusing. Rates of self-reported food allergy vary widely, and reach implausibly high numbers in small studies of varying methodologic rigor. In the sparse data that come from studies using food challenge, there are hints that less industrialized (or "Westernized") countries such as Thailand and Turkey may have lower rates of food allergy, but many of these studies only examined a select set of foods and may have other methodologic concerns. One of the most rigorously designed studies, the HealthNuts study, found the highest rate of confirmed allergy, primarily attributable to very high rates of egg allergy in infancy.[10] We discuss the potential reasons for this finding in the section on egg allergy. Examining prevalence trends for specific foods may give more insight into geographic differences in prevalence and the environmental exposures that contribute to food allergy.

Prevalence of Specific Food Allergies

In the United States, the most prevalent food allergies are to peanut, cow's milk, hen's egg, shellfish, tree nuts, wheat, fish, and soy. These 8 allergens are estimated to account for 90% of systemic food allergies in the United States.[28] Here we explore the epidemiology of peanut, tree nut, hen's egg, cow's milk, shellfish, and fish allergy because these are the foods to which allergy is both most common and most likely to involve serious reactions.

Peanut allergy

Peanut allergy is a major cause of food-related anaphylaxis. Most peanut allergy presents early in life, and most peanut allergic children do not outgrow their peanut allergy.[29] The prevalence of peanut allergy by self-report in the United States varies from about 1.2% to 2% in US children and 0.6% to 0.8% in US adults, with the higher rates in children thought to represent secular trends in peanut allergy rather than resolution of allergy.[3,4,8] Similar rates of self-reported peanut allergy were reported in various surveys in Western Europe and Canada, although, in general, rates of self-reported peanut allergy are higher in Northern Europe,[30] with low rates reported in the Middle East and Asia.[22,31–34] In Europe, a metaanalysis of peanut allergy prevalence put the rate of challenge confirmed peanut allergy much lower (0.2%), but this number increased to 1.6% when food challenge and history of peanut reactions were combined.[30] Investigation of the low prevalence of peanut allergy in Israel led to the hypothesis that early introduction of peanut prevents peanut allergy, a finding now confirmed in a randomized, controlled trial.[33] A relative dearth of peanut allergy in East and Central Asian countries is potentially secondary to dietary or environmental differences, particularly the form of peanut consumed (boiled vs roasted).[35]

Tree nut allergy

The tree nuts include, but are not limited to, walnut, pecan, hazelnut, cashew, pistachio, almond, pine nut, and Brazil nuts. The natural history of tree nut allergy is distinct from most other foods, with prevalence increasing over time and resolution a relatively rare occurrence (<20%).[36] Tree nut allergy is also unusual in that a substantial proportion of tree nut allergy falls within the category of OAS. Notwithstanding OAS, tree nut allergy is one of the most common causes of anaphylaxis, accounting for up to 40% of cases in some series,[37] and, together with peanut allergy, up to 90% of food-related fatalities.

In the United States, most estimates of the prevalence of tree nut allergy are around 1%.[3,4,8] Recently, McWilliam and associates[37] performed a systematic review of the prevalence of tree nut allergy worldwide. Among the 7 studies that used oral food challenge, the prevalence in children was 0% to 1.4%, whereas 0% to 4.9% reported tree nut allergy, and 0.8% to 6.5% were sensitized to at least 1 tree nut. No studies of adults were done that used oral food challenge, but self-reported rates ranged from 0.18% to 8.9%. Generally, studies from Europe showed a higher prevalence of tree nut allergy, a finding thought to be related to the patterns of pollen allergy there, particularly birch allergy, and the concomitant OAS, but there are no data on the prevalence outside of North America, Asia, and Europe.[37]

In terms of individual tree nuts, hazelnut allergy was the most common food allergy reported in outpatient clinics in the EuroPrevall study, and was strongly associated with birch pollen allergy.[38] In the United States, walnut and cashew allergy seem to be the most common tree nut allergies, and in the UK, Brazil nut, almond, and walnut allergies are the most common.[37]

Egg allergy

Our understanding of egg allergy has become more nuanced in recent years, as we have come to understand that many children with egg allergy are able to tolerate extensively heated forms of egg.[39] Larger studies do not usually distinguish between these phenotypes.

In the United States, surveys relying on self-report place the prevalence of egg allergy among all children at 0.6% to 0.8% overall, at 1% among those 0 to 2 years of age, and at 0.5% among adults.[3,8] The overall rate of egg allergy in the

EuroPREVALL birth cohort, which used oral food challenges, is similar, with 1.2% of 1- to 2-year-old children estimated to have an egg allergy. Within this cohort, Northwestern European countries had the highest prevalence and Mediterranean and Eastern European countries the lowest, with differences greater than 200% between some countries (ie, Greece with a rate of 0.1% and the UK, with a rate of 2.2%).[40] However, a population-based study of 1-year-old children in Australia that used oral food challenges (HealthNuts) estimated the rate at 9%,[10] far higher than in any European country.

What can we make of the sky-high rates of egg allergy in Australia? It is possible that environmental or genetic differences may underlie these geographic variations, but it seems unlikely that either the genetic backgrounds of studied subjects or possible environmental risk factors (such as dietary practices, antibiotic use, etc) are so different between Australia and the United States or Europe. More likely, the ascertainment methods are to blame for these differences. In HealthNuts, all children were evaluated with egg skin prick testing, with those with a positive test offered an oral challenge with a raw egg powder, regardless of reported tolerance or reactivity. In contrast, in EuroPREVALL, it was only those with eczema or suspected egg allergy who were evaluated for sensitization, and only those who did not have a history of tolerating egg who were offered food challenge.[40] Given that 80% of those with egg allergy in HealthNuts tolerated baked egg,[10] and that the vast majority of egg allergy resolved by 4 years of age,[41] it is likely that many of the egg allergic cases identified in the HealthNuts study would not have ever been diagnosed with egg allergy outside of the study. The surprising take away is that underrecognition of food allergy may be as much of a factor as overreporting.

Milk allergy

There are several factors that make estimating the prevalence of milk allergy uniquely difficult. Most important is the spectrum of intolerances and allergies that are commonly caused by cow's milk exposure. Age-related lactase deficiency, which can lead to lactose intolerance, is reported to occur in up to 70% of the world's population,[42] and is often confused for allergy. Non–IgE-mediated allergic reactions to milk are also common, including allergic proctocolitis, which presents early in infancy.[43] In addition, like egg allergy, the epidemiology of milk allergy is confusing because most allergy resolves early in life, and because most people with IgE-mediated milk allergy are able to tolerate extensively heated milk.[44]

In the United States, about 2% of children and 2.6% of adults report a milk allergy.[3,8] A European metaanalysis in 2014 estimated the point prevalence of self-reported milk allergy to be 2%, and 0.6% for food challenge confirmed allergy.[30] Similarly, in a more recent report of the EuroPrevall birth cohorts, the overall cumulative incidence of food challenge proven cow's milk allergy was 0.5% in young children, with rates varying from less than 0.3% in Lithuania, Germany, and Greece, to 1% in the Netherlands and the UK.[44] In China, the self-reported rate of cow's milk allergy among kindergarteners was 1.9%,[45] with other studies in Hong Kong[31] and South Korea[46] finding milk allergy to be among the most commonly reported allergies. In contrast, a study of Turkish infants found a rate of only 0.1%,[47] but it was a relatively small study.

As with egg allergy, it seems that the rate of milk allergy is less in Southern than Northern Europe, but there are very few global data outside the United States and Europe.

Shellfish allergy

Shellfish are a group of foods to which individuals may be individually or multiply reactive, and include both mollusks (ie, squid, clams, and octopus) and crustaceans (ie, crab, shrimp, and lobster). In general, shellfish allergy tends to be persistent and to present later in life than many other food allergies. Crustaceans and mollusks share some cross-reactive proteins (most notably tropomyosin proteins), but crustacean allergy tends to be more common, and the majority of those with crustacean allergy can tolerate mollusks.[48]

The prevalence of any self-reported shellfish allergy among US children ranges from 0.5% to 2.0%,[3,8,48] whereas in Europe estimates of crustacean allergy range from 0.1% in Lithuania to 5.5% in France, and mollusk allergy from 0.5% in Portugal to 1.5% in France.[49] In Asia, there is a wide range of reported crustacean allergy among children, from 0.5% in Thailand[50] to 4.0% in Taiwan,[51] with fewer data about mollusk allergy. Among adults, self-reported prevalence of shellfish allergy in the United States is around 2.0% (2.0% in NHANES[8] and 2.5% in a telephone survey[48]). Worldwide, there are fewer data on adults, with an estimate of 2.0% allergic to shrimp in Denmark[27] and 3.3% in Taiwan.[51] There are few studies that have used food challenges to confirm allergy: in Denmark none of those younger than 3 years of age and 0.3% of adults had shrimp allergy, compared with 0.3% and 0.9% in 2 studies of children in Thailand.[21,27]

On the whole, the prevalence of shellfish allergy seems to be higher in adults than children, and may be higher in Asia, but more data are needed.

Fish allergy

Fish also encompass a wide range of foods, with variable cross-reactivity between species. Epidemiologic studies typically use cod as the prototypical fish or do not differentiate between species. The rate of self-reported fish allergy among children in the United States is relatively low, at 0.2% in a telephone survey[48] and 0.43% in NHANES,[8] whereas in Europe and the Middle East the self-reported rate ranges from 0% in Israel to 9% in Finland,[49] and in Asia, rates ranged from 0.2% in Hong Kong to 4.3% in the Phillipines.[49] In European studies confirming diagnosis with food challenge, the rate of fish allergy in children was 0.2% or less in Denmark,[27] Turkey,[52] the UK,[14] Thailand,[21] and Finland,[53] and 0.3% or less in adults in Denmark[27] and Turkey.[52] Thus, the overall prevalence of fish allergy seems to be low, except perhaps in certain specific countries.

CHANGES OVER TIME IN FOOD ALLERGY

Survey data in the United States clearly show an increase in the prevalence of self-reported food allergy in general, and peanut allergy in particular, among children over the past several decades. In a metaregression of studies sponsored by the Centers for Disease Control and Prevention, the estimated increase in food allergy prevalence was 1.2% per decade, such that the rates estimated by the National Health Interview Survey increased from 3.4% in 2000% to 4.6% in 2010.[54] Similarly, in the survey of peanut allergy conducted by Sicherer and colleagues,[4] the rate increased from 0.4% in 1997% to 1.4% in 2008.

Health care use for food allergy has also increased over the same period. In Illinois, there was an increase in food allergy-related visits to the emergency department and hospitalizations from 6.3 per 100,000 children in 2008 to 17.2 per 100,000 in 2012.[55] In Olmstead, Minnesota, estimates of peanut allergy from chart review increased from 0.2% to 0.7% between 1999 and 2007.[56] In the UK, an increase of 500% in food-related hospitalizations between 1990 and 2004 was seen,[57] whereas in Australia, hospital admissions for food-related anaphylaxis increased by 10% per year between 1997 and 2013.[58] Despite the clear increase in emergency department visits and hospitalizations for food allergy, the data on fatal food reactions are mixed.

Food allergy–related fatalities remained stable or even decreased in the UK, the United States, Brazil, and Canada during the same period that hospitalizations increased.[59–61] It is only in Australia where food allergy–related fatal reactions have increased during this time.[58] Interestingly, in that study, the vast majority of fatal reactions to foods occurred in individuals older than 20 years of age, and reactions to shellfish accounted for one-half of the fatalities.

In contrast with the striking increase in the prevalence of food allergy reflected in self-reported data and health care use, birth cohorts in the Isle of Wight in the UK established in 1989 and 2001 did not show changes in peanut allergy over time.[62] Even more surprising, comparison of IgE sensitization to milk, egg, and peanut in stored blood from children in NHANES III (collected between 1988 and 1994) with samples from NHANES 2005 to 2006 did not show any differences in rates of sensitization to those foods, which were high in both surveys. Indeed, shrimp sensitization actually decreased significantly between the surveys.[63]

Thus, although there is overwhelming evidence for increased perceived and diagnosed food allergy over the past several decades, the sparse data that we have from objective measures such as fatal reactions and IgE sensitization generally conflict with that trend. To understand whether changes are due to greater recognition or to other environmental changes, we need high-quality studies that incorporate objective measures with clinical data and are done repeatedly over time. Unfortunately, these kinds of studies require both foresight and significant resources.

SPECIFIC RISK POPULATIONS
Disparities Between African American and Other Racial Ethnic Groups in Food Allergy

Very significant racial and ethnic disparities in other allergic diseases, such as asthma, have long been noted, with African American children and adults experiencing much higher rates of asthma and asthma complications than white, Hispanic, or Asian children and adults.[64,65] There are fewer data about food allergy, but what is currently available suggests significant differences in sensitization to foods between racial and ethnic groups in the United States and in several other Westernized countries. Whether these sensitization differences are accompanied by differences in clinical food allergy is less clear.

In the NHANES 2005 to 2006 survey, the survey that included measurement of food specific IgE, non-Hispanic Black subjects were nearly twice as likely to be sensitized to food as non-Hispanic white subjects, and 27% more likely than Hispanic subjects.[7] Other, localized studies have also found higher rates of sensitization to foods among African American children, including in a Boston birth cohort,[66] a Michigan birth cohort,[67] and in an academic allergy practice in New York City.[68] Non–nationally representative cohorts of various groups, including those attending allergy clinics in New York, Chicago, and Cincinnati,[68] and those enrolled in a high-risk inner-city birth cohort,[69] have also suggested very high rates of food allergy among at least some African American pediatric populations. However, national data drawn from health care use data and self-reported surveys show a more complicated story.

Analyses of New York State hospital admissions, the National Hospital Ambulatory Medical Care Survey, and the National Electronic Injury Surveillance System found no significant racial or ethnic disparities in emergency room visits or hospitalizations for food allergy in years collectively spanning 1990 to 2006,[70–73] although there were more emergency room visits for anaphylaxis among African American children in Florida between 2005 and 2006.[74] Interestingly, in the yearly National Health Interview Survey, food allergy was reported in non-Hispanic African American children at rates less than or equal to that reported by non-Hispanic white children until the mid-2000s, when reported rates among African American children began to consistently exceed that of other ethnic groups.[54]

Thus, although sensitization to foods is higher among African American children, self-reported food allergy has only recently become more prevalent in this group. This is not likely due to increasing sensitization, because non-Hispanic Black children had higher levels of food-specific IgE in both NHANES III (collected between 1988 and 1994) and the later NHANES 2005 to 2006 data than other racial and ethnic groups, and there were no significant changes over time in any racial or ethnic group.[63] Interestingly, in NHANES III, it was only non-Hispanic white subjects who had a relationship between IgE sensitization to foods and reported history of acute reactions to food, suggesting at least an historical difference by race and ethnicity in the relationship between sensitization and perceived allergy.[6] Although these results suggest that historically African American children had less recognition of food allergy, it is possible that these findings represent true differences in the relationship between IgE and clinical allergy. More, and more recent, data are needed to truly understand racial and ethnic disparities in food allergy.

Role of Immigration on Food Allergy Rates

It is not only African American children who seem to have particularly high rates of food allergy. In the United States and Australia, children of immigrants from less developed countries are noted to have a higher risk of food allergy than either children of native-born populations or immigrants themselves. In Australia, children with Asian-born mothers had more than twice the odds of nut allergy compared with non-Asian children, whereas those born in Asia had 10 times less nut allergy.[75] In the United States, children of immigrants had a 50% higher odds of food sensitization than children of nonimmigrants, even accounting for race and ethnicity, whereas those who were born outside the United States had a 50% lower odds.[76] It is likely that these findings are due to gene-by-environment interactions that leave some children with specific genetic backgrounds more at risk for allergy development under specific environmental conditions found in Western countries. More research is needed to identify causal genetic and environmental factors that drive these differences.

SUMMARY

Food allergy is a highly prevalent problem. There is some evidence that food allergy prevalence is increasing, although the data to support this trend are mixed. Geographic and temporal differences in food allergy prevalence suggest the importance of environmental factors in the development of food allergy. More research is needed to identify the most important factors.

REFERENCES

1. Winberg A, West CE, Strinnholm A, et al. Assessment of allergy to milk, egg, cod, and wheat in Swedish schoolchildren: a population based cohort study. PLoS One 2015;10(7):e0131804.
2. McGowan EC, Matsui EC, Peng R, et al. Racial/ethnic and socioeconomic differences in self-reported food allergy among food-sensitized children in National Health and Nutrition Examination Survey III. Ann Allergy Asthma Immunol 2016; 117(5):570–2.e3.

3. Gupta RS, Springston EE, Warrier MR, et al. The prevalence, severity, and distribution of childhood food allergy in the united states. Pediatrics 2011;128(1): e9–17.

4. Sicherer SH, Munoz-Furlong A, Godbold JH, et al. US prevalence of self-reported peanut, tree nut, and sesame allergy: 11-year follow-up. J Allergy Clin Immunol 2010;125(6):1322–6.

5. Soller L, Ben-Shoshan M, Harrington DW, et al. Adjusting for nonresponse bias corrects overestimates of food allergy prevalence. J Allergy Clin Immunol Pract 2015;3(2):291–3.e2.

6. McGowan EC, Matsui EC, McCormack MC, et al. Effect of poverty, urbanization, and race/ethnicity on perceived food allergy in the United States. Ann Allergy Asthma Immunol 2015;115(1):85–6.e2.

7. Liu AH, Jaramillo R, Sicherer SH, et al. National prevalence and risk factors for food allergy and relationship to asthma: results from the National Health and Nutrition Examination Survey 2005-2006. J Allergy Clin Immunol 2010;126(4): 798–806.e13.

8. McGowan EC, Keet CA. Prevalence of self-reported food allergy in the National Health and Nutrition Examination Survey (NHANES) 2007-2010. J Allergy Clin Immunol 2013;132(5):1216–9.e5.

9. Mills EN, Mackie AR, Burney P, et al. The prevalence, cost and basis of food allergy across Europe. Allergy 2007;62(7):717–22.

10. Osborne NJ, Koplin JJ, Martin PE, et al. Prevalence of challenge-proven IgE-mediated food allergy using population-based sampling and predetermined challenge criteria in infants. J Allergy Clin Immunol 2011;127(3):668–76.e1-2.

11. Katelaris CH. Food allergy and oral allergy or pollen-food syndrome. Curr Opin Allergy Clin Immunol 2010;10(3):246–51.

12. Venter C, Pereira B, Grundy J, et al. Incidence of parentally reported and clinically diagnosed food hypersensitivity in the first year of life. J Allergy Clin Immunol 2006;117(5):1118–24.

13. Venter C, Pereira B, Voigt K, et al. Prevalence and cumulative incidence of food hypersensitivity in the first 3 years of life. Allergy 2008;63(3):354–9.

14. Venter C, Pereira B, Grundy J, et al. Prevalence of sensitization reported and objectively assessed food hypersensitivity amongst six-year-old children: a population-based study. Pediatr Allergy Immunol 2006;17(5):356–63.

15. Eller E, Kjaer HF, Host A, et al. Development of atopic dermatitis in the DARC birth cohort. Pediatr Allergy Immunol 2010;21(2 Pt 1):307–14.

16. US Department of Health and Human Services, Centers for Disease Control and Prevention, National Center for Health Statistics. Summary statistics, national health interview survey 2015, table C-2A. 2015.

17. Branum AM, Simon AE, Lukacs SL. Among children with food allergy, do socio-demographic factors and healthcare use differ by severity? Matern Child Health J 2012;16(Suppl 1):S44–50.

18. Verrill L, Bruns R, Luccioli S. Prevalence of self-reported food allergy in U.S. adults: 2001, 2006, and 2010. Allergy Asthma Proc 2015;36(6):458–67.

19. Prescott SL, Pawankar R, Allen KJ, et al. A global survey of changing patterns of food allergy burden in children. World Allergy Organ J 2013;6(1):21.

20. Burney P, Summers C, Chinn S, et al. Prevalence and distribution of sensitization to foods in the European Community Respiratory Health Survey: a EuroPrevall analysis. Allergy 2010;65(9):1182–8.

21. Lao-Araya M, Trakultivakorn M. Prevalence of food allergy among preschool children in northern Thailand. Pediatr Int 2012;54(2):238–43.

22. Chen J, Hu Y, Allen KJ, et al. The prevalence of food allergy in infants in Chongqing, China. Pediatr Allergy Immunol 2011;22(4):356–60.
23. Grimshaw KEC, Bryant T, Oliver EM, et al. Incidence and risk factors for food hypersensitivity in UK infants: results from a birth cohort study. Clin Transl Allergy 2016;6(1):1.
24. Mustafayev R, Civelek E, Orhan F, et al. Similar prevalence, different spectrum: IgE-mediated food allergy among Turkish adolescents. Allergol Immunopathol (Madr) 2013;41(6):387–96.
25. Kjaer HF, Eller E, Host A, et al. The prevalence of allergic diseases in an unselected group of 6-year-old children. the DARC birth cohort study. Pediatr Allergy Immunol 2008;19(8):737–45.
26. Venter C, Hasan Arshad S, Grundy J, et al. Time trends in the prevalence of peanut allergy: three cohorts of children from the same geographical location in the UK. Allergy 2010;65(1):103–8.
27. Osterballe M, Hansen TK, Mortz CG, et al. The prevalence of food hypersensitivity in an unselected population of children and adults. Pediatr Allergy Immunol 2005;16(7):567–73.
28. Food allergen labeling and consumer protection act of 2004. 2004;108–202:202.
29. Skolnick HS, Conover-Walker MK, Koerner CB, et al. The natural history of peanut allergy. J Allergy Clin Immunol 2001;107(2):367–74.
30. Nwaru BI, Hickstein L, Panesar SS, et al. Prevalence of common food allergies in Europe: a systematic review and meta-analysis. Allergy 2014;69(8):992–1007.
31. Ho MH, Lee SL, Wong WH, et al. Prevalence of self-reported food allergy in Hong Kong children and teens–a population survey. Asian Pac J Allergy Immunol 2012; 30(4):275–84.
32. Kaya A, Erkocoglu M, Civelek E, et al. Prevalence of confirmed IgE-mediated food allergy among adolescents in turkey. Pediatr Allergy Immunol 2013;24(5): 456–62.
33. Du Toit G, Roberts G, Sayre PH, et al. Randomized trial of peanut consumption in infants at risk for peanut allergy. N Engl J Med 2015;372(9):803–13.
34. Orhan F, Karakas T, Cakir M, et al. Prevalence of immunoglobulin E-mediated food allergy in 6-9-year-old urban schoolchildren in the eastern black sea region of turkey. Clin Exp Allergy 2009;39(7):1027–35.
35. Arakali SR, Green TD, Dinakar C. Prevalence of food allergies in south Asia. Ann Allergy Asthma Immunol 2017;118(1):16–20.
36. Fleischer DM, Conover-Walker MK, Matsui EC, et al. The natural history of tree nut allergy. J Allergy Clin Immunol 2005;116(5):1087–93.
37. McWilliam V, Koplin J, Lodge C, et al. The prevalence of tree nut allergy: a systematic review. Curr Allergy Asthma Rep 2015;15(9):54.
38. Datema MR, Zuidmeer-Jongejan L, Asero R, et al. Hazelnut allergy across Europe dissected molecularly: a EuroPrevall outpatient clinic survey. J Allergy Clin Immunol 2015;136(2):382–91.
39. Tey D, Heine RG. Egg allergy in childhood: an update. Curr Opin Allergy Clin Immunol 2009;9(3):244–50.
40. Xepapadaki P, Fiocchi A, Grabenhenrich L, et al. Incidence and natural history of hen's egg allergy in the first 2 years of life-the EuroPrevall birth cohort study. Allergy 2016;71(3):350–7.
41. Peters RL, Koplin JJ, Gurrin LC, et al. The prevalence of food allergy and other allergic diseases in early childhood in a population-based study: HealthNuts age 4-year follow-up. J Allergy Clin Immunol 2017;140(1):145–53.e8.

42. Corgneau M, Scher J, Ritie-Pertusa L, et al. Recent advances on lactose intolerance: tolerance thresholds and currently available answers. Crit Rev Food Sci Nutr 2017;57(15):3344–56.

43. Feuille E, Nowak-Wegrzyn A. Food protein-induced enterocolitis syndrome, allergic proctocolitis, and enteropathy. Curr Allergy Asthma Rep 2015;15(8):50.

44. Schoemaker AA, Sprikkelman AB, Grimshaw KE, et al. Incidence and natural history of challenge-proven cow's milk allergy in European children–EuroPrevall birth cohort. Allergy 2015;70(8):963–72.

45. Zeng GQ, Luo JY, Huang HM, et al. Food allergy and related risk factors in 2540 preschool children: an epidemiological survey in Guangdong province, southern China. World J Pediatr 2015;11(3):219–25.

46. Park M, Kim D, Ahn K, et al. Prevalence of immediate-type food allergy in early childhood in seoul. Allergy Asthma Immunol Res 2014;6(2):131–6.

47. Zeyrek D, Koruk I, Kara B, et al. Prevalence of IgE mediated cow's milk and egg allergy in children under 2 years of age in Sanliurfa, Turkey: the city that isn't almost allergic to cow's milk. Minerva Pediatr 2015;67(6):465–72.

48. Sicherer SH, Munoz-Furlong A, Sampson HA. Prevalence of seafood allergy in the united states determined by a random telephone survey. J Allergy Clin Immunol 2004;114(1):159–65.

49. Moonesinghe H, Mackenzie H, Venter C, et al. Prevalence of fish and shellfish allergy: a systematic review. Ann Allergy Asthma Immunol 2016;117(3):264–72.e4.

50. Santadusit S, Atthapaisalsarudee S, Vichyanond P. Prevalence of adverse food reactions of adverse food reactions and food allergy among Thai children. J Med Assoc Thai 2005;88(Supplement 8):S31.

51. Wu TC, Tsai TC, Huang CF, et al. Prevalence of food allergy in Taiwan: a questionnaire-based survey. Intern Med J 2012;42(12):1310–5.

52. Gelincik A, Buyukozturk S, Gul H, et al. Confirmed prevalence of food allergy and non-allergic food hypersensitivity in a Mediterranean population. Clin Exp Allergy 2008;38(8):1333–41.

53. Kajosaari M. Food allergy in finish children aged 1 to 6 years. Acta Paediatr Scand 1982;71(5):815–9.

54. Keet CA, Savage JH, Seopaul S, et al. Temporal trends and racial/ethnic disparity in self-reported pediatric food allergy in the united states. Ann Allergy Asthma Immunol 2014;112(3):222–9.e3.

55. Dyer AA, Lau CH, Smith TL, et al. Pediatric emergency department visits and hospitalizations due to food-induced anaphylaxis in Illinois. Ann Allergy Asthma Immunol 2015;115(1):56–62.

56. Rinaldi M, Harnack L, Oberg C, et al. Peanut allergy diagnoses among children residing in Olmsted County, Minnesota. J Allergy Clin Immunol 2012;130(4):945–50.

57. Turner PJ, Gowland MH, Sharma V, et al. Increase in anaphylaxis-related hospitalizations but no increase in fatalities: an analysis of united kingdom national anaphylaxis data, 1992-2012. J Allergy Clin Immunol 2015;135(4):956–63.e1.

58. Mullins RJ, Wainstein BK, Barnes EH, et al. Increases in anaphylaxis fatalities in Australia from 1997 to 2013. Clin Exp Allergy 2016;46(8):1099–110.

59. Ma L, Danoff TM, Borish L. Case fatality and population mortality associated with anaphylaxis in the united states. J Allergy Clin Immunol 2014;133(4):1075–83.

60. Tanno LK, Ganem F, Demoly P, et al. Undernotification of anaphylaxis deaths in brazil due to difficult coding under the ICD-10. Allergy 2012;67(6):783–9.

61. Jerschow E, Lin RY, Scaperotti MM, et al. Fatal anaphylaxis in the united states, 1999-2010: temporal patterns and demographic associations. J Allergy Clin Immunol 2014;134(6):1318–28.e7.
62. Venter C, Maslin K, Patil V, et al. The prevalence, natural history and time trends of peanut allergy over the first 10 years of life in two cohorts born in the same geographical location 12 years apart. Pediatr Allergy Immunol 2016;27(8): 804–11.
63. McGowan EC, Peng RD, Salo PM, et al. Changes in food-specific IgE over time in the National Health and Nutrition Examination Survey (NHANES). J Allergy Clin Immunol Pract 2016;4(4):713–20.
64. Keet CA, Matsui EC, McCormack MC, et al. Urban residence, neighborhood poverty, race/ethnicity, and asthma morbidity among children on Medicaid. J Allergy Clin Immunol 2017;140(3):822–7.
65. Keet CA, McCormack MC, Pollack CE, et al. Neighborhood poverty, urban residence, race/ethnicity, and asthma: rethinking the inner-city asthma epidemic. J Allergy Clin Immunol 2015;135(3):655–62.
66. Kumar R, Tsai HJ, Hong X, et al. Race, ancestry, and development of food-allergen sensitization in early childhood. Pediatrics 2011;128(4):e821–9.
67. Joseph CL, Zoratti EM, Ownby DR, et al. Exploring racial differences in IgE-mediated food allergy in the WHEALS birth cohort. Ann Allergy Asthma Immunol 2016;116(3):219–24.e1.
68. Taylor-Black S, Wang J. The prevalence and characteristics of food allergy in urban minority children. Ann Allergy Asthma Immunol 2012;109(6):431–7.
69. Mahdavinia M, Fox SR, Smith BM, et al. Racial differences in food allergy phenotype and health care utilization among US children. J Allergy Clin Immunol Pract 2017;5(2):352–7.e1.
70. Lin RY, Anderson AS, Shah SN, et al. Increasing anaphylaxis hospitalizations in the first 2 decades of life: New York state, 1990 -2006. Ann Allergy Asthma Immunol 2008;101(4):387–93.
71. Rudders SA, Espinola JA, Camargo CA Jr. North-south differences in US emergency department visits for acute allergic reactions. Ann Allergy Asthma Immunol 2010;104(5):413–6.
72. Ross MP, Ferguson M, Street D, et al. Analysis of food-allergic and anaphylactic events in the national electronic injury surveillance system. J Allergy Clin Immunol 2008;121(1):166–71.
73. Greenhawt M, Weiss C, Conte ML, et al. Racial and ethnic disparity in food allergy in the united states: a systematic review. J Allergy Clin Immunol Pract 2013;1(4): 378–86.
74. Harduar-Morano L, Simon MR, Watkins S, et al. A population-based epidemiologic study of emergency department visits for anaphylaxis in Florida. J Allergy Clin Immunol 2011;128(3):594–600.e1.
75. Panjari M, Koplin JJ, Dharmage SC, et al. Nut allergy prevalence and differences between Asian-born children and Australian-born children of Asian descent: a state-wide survey of children at primary school entry in Victoria, Australia. Clin Exp Allergy 2016;46(4):602–9.
76. Keet CA, Wood RA, Matsui EC. Personal and parental nativity as risk factors for food sensitization. J Allergy Clin Immunol 2012;129(1):169–75.e1-5.

Oral Tolerance Development and Maintenance

Erik Wambre, PhD[a],*, David Jeong, MD[b]

KEYWORDS

- Food allergy • Immune tolerance • Microbiome • Mucosal immunity
- Immunotherapy • CD4$^+$ T cells • Dendritic cells

KEY POINTS

- The gastrointestinal tract has an abundant mucosal immune system to develop and maintain oral tolerance.
- The oral route of administration takes advantage of the unique set of immune cells and pathways involved in the induction of oral tolerance.
- Food allergy results from a loss of oral tolerance toward ingested antigens.
- Oral immunotherapy is thought to initiate desensitization through interaction of an allergen with mucosal dendritic cells that initiate downstream immune system modulation through regulatory T cells and effector T cells.

INTRODUCTION

Tolerance is the the ability to endure what one cannot avoid and is also referred to as an accepted dispensation to particular rules. When applied to orally administrated antigen, the definition of tolerance represents the capacity of the immune system to adapt to innocuous dietary proteins and commensal bacteria because we are unable to avoid them. These antigens are detected in the gut epithelium and lamina propria (LP) within minutes after consumption,[1] suggesting a critical role of the gastrointestinal (GI) tract in oral tolerance development. Currently, it is postulated that this state of unresponsiveness to ingested antigens is initiated by tolerogenic CD103 + DCs residing in the GI LP.[2] Following capture of luminal antigens, these cells migrate to the draining lymph node to present antigen-derived epitopes to induce antigen-specific regulatory CD4 + T cells. Failure to develop oral tolerance can lead to a cascade of adverse reactions such as immunoglobulin E (IgE)-mediated food allergies, celiac disease, autoimmune diseases, and infections. These immune-related disorders have emerged as

[a] Benaroya Research Institute at Virginia Mason, 1201 Ninth Avenue, Seattle, WA 98101, USA;
[b] Virginia Mason Medical Center, 1201 Terry Avenue, Seattle, WA 98101, USA
* Corresponding author.
E-mail address: ewambre@benaroyaresearch.org

Immunol Allergy Clin N Am 38 (2018) 27–37
https://doi.org/10.1016/j.iac.2017.09.003
0889-8561/18/© 2017 Elsevier Inc. All rights reserved.

immunology.theclinics.com

major health problems worldwide because of the rapid increase in prevalence over the past decade.[3] Food-induced allergic reactions are an immediate, adverse reaction triggered predominantly by cross-linking of food-derived antigen-specific IgE bound to the high-affinity IgE receptor FcεR on mast cells after reexposure to allergen.[4,5] These allergic reactions can cause clinical symptoms ranging from mild mouth itching and abdominal pain to life-threatening anaphylaxis. Standard of care is allergen avoidance and prompt treatment of allergic reactions when they develop after accidental ingestion. One promising area of current investigation is the use of oral immunotherapy (OIT) as a method to eventually restore oral tolerance to food. Improving the understanding of oral tolerance mechanisms will aid in the reduction of food allergy prevalence rates through preexposure prophylaxis (due to natural tolerance development) and create new strategies for food allergy therapy (due to induced tolerance).

THE GASTROINTESTINAL MUCOSA: A UNIQUE PLACE IN ORAL TOLERANCE DEVELOPMENT

The GI tract is exposed to a large array of non-self-antigen on a continual basis, including numerous commensal bacteria and well over 30 kg of food proteins per year.[6] Nevertheless, the GI immune system does not elicit cellular or humoral immune responses to these harmless antigens because it protects against pathogenic microbes. This phenomenon of balancing the immune response to commensal microbes and food has been termed "oral tolerance" and refers to local and systemic immune unresponsiveness to orally administered soluble antigens. It may develop naturally or be induced by allergen immunotherapy. The GI mucosa is the largest immunologic site in the body designed to distinguish between beneficial and harmful components in the gut to maintain systemic immune tolerance.[7,8] It is composed of 3 major compartments: the epithelial layer, the LP, and the gut-associated lymphoid tissue (GALT), where adaptive immune responses are initiated.[9] Immune responses in the gut are efficiently induced in mesenteric lymph nodes (mLN) and Peyer patches (PP), which are the main components of the organized GALT. PPs are lymphoid-cell accumulation areas found in the submucosa, primarily the small intestine, and consist of B-cell follicles and surrounding T-cell areas. Intestinal epithelial cells form a tight and selective barrier that allows highly controlled paracellular and transcellular transport of molecules or antigens necessary to the induction of appropriate immune responses in the gut.[10] The barrier function of the GI tract is aided by the presence of a protective, hydrophobic mucus-coated surface that traps antigen and dimeric IgA that binds food proteins. Together this prevents absorption of antigen across the intestinal epithelium.[11] However, an estimated 2% of gut luminal food proteins pass through the gut epithelium intact and are disseminated locally or systemically through the circulation or the lymphatic system.[12] Tissue-resident T lymphocytes are abundant in the GI immune system and play important roles in mucosal immunity and oral tolerance.[13] Their adaptation to these environments requires constant discrimination between natural stimulation coming from harmless microbiota and food, and pathogens that need to be cleared. Several factors are involved to ensure durable tolerance to harmless intestinally derived antigens, including the dose, nature, and routes of antigen entry at sensitization. Physical barriers, digestion, and composition of the intestinal flora are also thought to contribute to the ability to develop oral tolerance.[14] The microbiome is a complex collection of resident bacteria in the gut and elsewhere that can profoundly impact immune responses in the GI tract. For instance, gut microbiota has been associated with increased production of IgA that may protect against food allergy by neutralizing food antigens and limiting their access to the immune system.[15,16]

Exposing children to a variety of food types from an early age might be an important contributing factor to induction of oral immune tolerance, thus preventing the development of severe food allergies.[17,18]

MECHANISM OF ORAL TOLERANCE

Despite a growing literature in the field, mechanisms of how ingested protein are normally rendered nonimmunogenic through oral tolerance are not fully understood and largely rely on murine experimental models. The initial contact between immune cells and antigens from the lumen is a critical step in the induction of intestinal immune response. Hadis and colleagues[19] recently proposed a model of stepwise oral tolerance induction comprising the generation of Treg cells in the gut-draining lymph nodes, followed by migration into the gut and subsequent local expansion of Treg cells driven by intestinal macrophages. Upon ingestion, immunogenic food proteins are denatured and degraded into small peptides by the digestive process in the gut. Absorption and transport of the luminal antigen involve complex processes, which might include transcytosis through intestinal epithelial cells, paracellular diffusion, and endocytosis via microfold cells (M cells), thus enabling antigenic presentation to underlying immune cells. Dendritic cells (DCs) that express the integrin CD11b and the chemokine receptor CX3CR1 can also directly sample the luminal content through the formation of transepithelial dendrites.[20–22] In specific areas of the epithelium, called PPs, internalized luminal antigens are captured by antigen-presenting cells, which then migrate into gut-draining mLN where they initiate activation and differentiation of effector or regulatory T cells (Treg) depending on cytokine milieu.[23] In the LP, DCs that express the integrin CD103 and CD11c promote IgA production, imprint gut homing on lymphocytes, and promote the differentiation of naïve T cells into Treg cells.[2] Intestinal mucin and cytokines produced by epithelial cells and innate lymphoid cells may also contribute to tolerance by modifying the phenotype of GI DCs.[16,24] It is also postulated that a different type of epithelial cell, the goblet cell, preferentially delivers luminal antigen to tolerogenic DCs implying a key role for this cell in intestinal immune homeostasis.[25] Compared with CD103 + DCs, antigen-loaded CX3CR1+ DCs do not express CCR7 and thus do not migrate to the mLN. Their role seems to be restricted to the local antigen-specific expansion of Treg cells in the LP. Vitamin A metabolite retinoic acid, Indolemine 2,3-dioxygenase (IDO) interleukin-10 (IL-10), and transforming growth factor-beta (TGF-β) (all produced by CD103 + DC) are thought to be critical determinants in defining the mLN tolerogenic environment.[26,27] Following activation, T cells differentiated in mLN by CD103 + DC then upregulate the gut-homing molecules integrin α4β7 and the chemokine (C-C motif) receptor 9 (CCR9), which provides homing properties to the activated T cells to migrate back to the LP.[28,29] Treg cells then undergo expansion under the influence of IL-10 produced by local antigen-loaded CX3CR1+DC cells (**Fig. 1**). Although Treg cells specific to food allergens are formed and localized in the intestine, they also can be found in circulation to maintain systemic tolerance.[30]

For many years, oral immune tolerance was envisioned as a multifaceted process involving clonal deletion, clonal anergy of reactive T cells, and the active regulation by Treg cells. In this context, Weiner and colleagues[31,32] suggested that the mechanism of oral tolerance was determined by the feeding regime used, with single high doses of antigen favoring clonal deletion or anergy, whereas multiple low doses of antigen were linked to T-cell–mediated suppression. However, transfer of CD25 + CD4+ T cells (which include Foxp3 + Tregs and activated effector cells) can induce oral tolerance to naïve animals.[33] Similarly, depletion of antigen-specific FoxP3+ cells

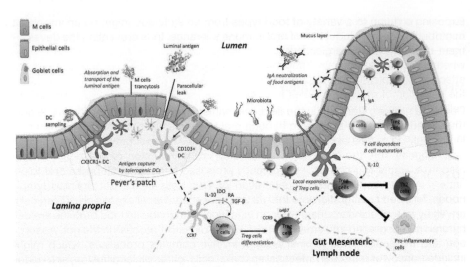

Fig. 1. Schematic overview of the stepwise mechanisms involved in the development and maintenance of oral tolerance. Upon ingestion and digestive process, luminal antigen is absorbed and transported through intestinal epithelial cells, thus enabling antigenic presentation to underlying immune cells. This complex process might include the following: (1) paracellular diffusion, (2) endocytosis via M cells and goblet cells, and (3) transepithelial DC sampling of the luminal antigen. In specific areas of the epithelium, called PPs, luminal antigens are taken up by CD11c + CD103 + DCs or CD11b + CX3CR1+DCs. Although CX3CR1+DCs remain located in the LP, antigen-loaded CD103 + DCs migrate to the mLN in a CCR7-dependent mechanism to promote the differentiation of naïve T cells into Treg cells. After their generation in lymph nodes, Tregs upregulate CCR9 and integrin α4β7 to home back to the LP where they undergo local expansion to induce oral tolerance. In this process Treg cells play a major role in the following: (1) promoting B-cell class switching to produce the noninflammatory IgA responses, (2) inducing T-cell anergy of effector cells, and (3) inhibiting downstream proinflammatory cells. RA, retinoic acid.

completely abolishes established functional oral tolerance, suggesting a dominant role of immunosuppressive FoxP3+ Treg cells in this process, especially Treg cells induced from conventional T cells in the periphery (pTreg cells).[34] Although there are multiple subtypes of pTregs,[8,9] both Foxp3+ and IL-10 producing Foxp3-pTregs are found in the GI tract. Their ability to produce pleiotropic immunoregulatory cytokines, such as TGF-β and IL-10, plays a major role in promoting B-cell class switching to produce the noninflammatory IgA responses. IL-10 also induces T-cell anergy of effector cells, sustains Treg populations, and directly participates in inhibiting downstream proinflammatory cells, such as mast cells, basophils, and eosinophils, leading to a state of unresponsiveness to ingested antigens or oral tolerance.[5,22]

Tolerance to intestinal bacteria and tolerance to food proteins differ by its effects on the immune system. However, it has been suggested that the presence of both diet- and microbiota-induced populations of pTreg cells may be required for complete tolerance to food antigens.[35,36] Using germ-free mice raised and bred on an elemental diet devoid of solid food dietary antigens, Kim and colleagues[37] recently demonstrated that the food antigens triggered FoxP3+ Treg cells to proliferate and accumulate in the small intestine LP, whereas microbiota elicit pTreg cell generation in the colon, implying that a carefully controlled process regulates the local expansion of pTreg cells. In this elegant study, the investigators also found that pTreg cells that suppress immune responses to food are phenotypically and functionally distinct from microbiota-induced RORγt + pTreg cells generated in the colon. However, food antigen–induced pTreg cells appear to have a relatively short lifespan, and it is unclear whether these food antigen–induced pTreg cells are also responsible for the systemic effects of oral tolerance. In experimental models of food allergy, it has been shown that the depletion of macromolecules from the diet precludes the development of pTreg cells in the small intestine.[38] In parallel, oral tolerance was maintained for several months after a single encounter with antigen, suggesting that the generation of pTregs in response to intestinal antigens might be a continuously ongoing process.[39]

LOSS OF ORAL TOLERANCE

Food allergy and celiac disease are the most prevalent food-induced pathology and are likely one of the consequences of a breakdown of oral tolerance characterized by elevated levels of IgE-positive myeloid cells (MC) in the small intestine.[40] How oral tolerance might be disrupted in food allergies remains unclear, but a weakened ability to induce or regenerate pTreg cells after exposure to food allergen may be a significant factor. For example, reduction in the number of pTreg cells has been documented in children with food allergy.[41] Failure to induce immunologic tolerance to food antigens is also thought to be affected by the timing of introduction to solid food, dose of antigen exposure, and allergenic property of the food themselves acting as mucosal TH2 adjuvants.[17] More recently, alterations in gut microflora composition have been implicated in the increase of allergy incidence. Gut microorganisms are the major source of natural antigens that continuously stimulate the GALT and induce mucosal immune tolerance to food proteins and molecular components of commensal bacteria.[42] Disruption of the microbiome can occur via early antibiotic use in infants and in utero, even with very low doses.[43] On occasion, these effects can persist well into adulthood.[44] A Western diet, typically high in fat but also low in fiber, may also be a critical determinant for intestinal flora diversity favoring or disfavoring Treg induction and epithelial integrity.[45] In a recent study, Tan and colleagues[46] established a role for dietary fiber in enhancing the tolerogenic CD103 + DC functions, suggesting that their phenotype is highly dependent on environmental conditioning factors present locally in the small intestine.[47]

The general immune mechanism behind allergic sensitization to food and thus of breakdown of oral tolerance can be viewed as a stepwise process initiated by disturbances in antigen uptake, dissemination, and/or presentation of allergen-derived epitope. Indeed, those with food allergy are thought to have genetic predisposition factors for higher skin and gut permeability as well as increasing allergen penetrance (which can be further exacerbated by environmental insults).[48] It is also increasingly understood that infants can become sensitized to foods through skin contact alone, particularly in those individuals with eczema who demonstrate loss of function filaggrin mutations.[49] Local disruption of the skin barrier integrity in the post–birth environment may condition mucosal DCs toward allergic sensitization versus the establishment of oral tolerance to ingested foods. For instance, presence of bacteria-induced barrier-protective response such as Clostridia in microbiota protects against sensitization by causing innate immune cells to produce high levels of IL-22, a signaling molecule known to decrease the permeability of the intestinal lining.[15] Conversely, intestinal inflammation can also abrogate the ability of CD103 + DCs to promote pTreg cell differentiation.[50] Thus, one can argue that allergic sensitization to food antigens via a damaged GI tract may confer susceptibility to food allergy later in life. In susceptible individuals, local tissue perturbations lead to increased concentration of epithelial-derived cytokine, such as IL-25, IL-33, and thymic stromal lymphopoietin (TSLP) at mucosal surfaces.[51] Acting through their respective receptors IL-17RB, ST2, and TSLP-R, the resultant type 2–permissive microenvironment instructs TH2 cell–mediated allergic inflammation through effects on DCs and on tissue-resident ILC2 cells. Among TH2 cells, the authors' group recently showed that allergen-specific TH2 cells represent a phenotypically distinct subset defined as CD4+ T cells that coexpress the surface molecule CRTH2, CD161, and CD49d, but lack CD27 and CD45RB expression.[52] In contrast to conventional TH2 cells, this proallergic TH2 subset (confined to atopic individuals) coexpressed IL-33-R and IL-25R,[52–54] providing evidence that food allergen-specific TH2 cell function may depend on tissue-derived cytokines at sites of tissue damage that regulate allergic immunity. Van Dyken and colleagues[55] further demonstrated that TH2 cells require stimulation by epithelial-derived cytokine in order to become functional TH2 effector cells in tissue, thereby comprising a checkpoint for effector cytokine acquisition. These findings validate the strategy of blocking tissue signals to treat allergic disease. Following allergic sensitization, proallergic TH2 cells migrate to a draining lymphoid node and prompt B cells to class switch, resulting in the production of IgE. IgE then binds to its high-affinity receptor FcεRI on the surface of mast cells and basophils, thereby arming these cells for activation.[56] After the occurrence of allergic sensitization, endogenous intestinal IL-25 produced constitutively by tuft cells, 1 of the 5 intestinal epithelial cell lineages, may rapidly establish a positive feedback loop that increases ILC2s and T_H2A effector functions. This TH2-permissive environment subsequently dampens the Treg cell population.[57,58] Atopic IL-4 signaling may also perpetuate allergic reactions to dietary proteins by inducing FcεR-expressing mast cell progenitors to develop into multifunctional IL-9-producing mucosal mast cells (MMC9s), which then expand greatly after repeated food ingestion.[59] These cells function as type-2–promoting innate MCs by generating prodigious amounts of the TH2 cytokines IL-9 and IL-13 and using mast cell function (via the secretion of histamine and proteases). Thus, it is possible that local accumulation of IgE-bearing MMC9s will impose the breakdown of oral tolerance to ingested food antigens, as recently reviewed by Wang.[24]

RESTORATION OF ORAL TOLERANCE DURING IMMUNOTHERAPY

Evidence of a lack of oral tolerance in food allergic patients has increased the interest in using OIT as a disease-modifying therapy via an effect on the gut immune system. The oral route of administration takes advantage of the unique properties of the intestinal immune system to induce tolerance. Such ability of continuous and gradual increase of orally administered antigen to restore oral tolerance to food allergens was first described in 1908 by A.T. Schofield.[60] At present, OIT is one of the most actively investigated therapeutic approaches for food allergy. However, in most cases, only patients remaining on maintenance doses do not develop reactions, and it is uncertain whether OIT leads to the development of oral tolerance or only to desensitization. Consumption of bacterial strains, such as Bifidobacterium longum 35624 and Clostridia, can result in increased numbers of intestinal Foxp3+ Treg cells that are capable of suppressing food allergy and colitis.[15,61] However, in the Nagler and colleagues study,[15] reintroduction of another major group of intestinal bacteria Bacteroides, failed to alleviate sensitization. Thus, one would envision that opportunistic intestinal flora is involved in the process of cultivating oral tolerance.

Immunologic changes accompanying oral desensitization include decreased reactivity of mast cells and basophils, increased food-specific IgG4 antibodies, and eventually decreased food-specific IgE antibodies.[62] OIT is thought to restore oral tolerance in patients with food allergy through interaction of the allergen with mucosal DC that initiates downstream immune system modulation through development of Treg cells.[63] For example, a higher frequency of milk allergen–specific Treg cells has been shown to correlate with a phenotype of mild clinical disease and favorable prognosis.[64] Desensitization is the first change noted with the initiation of OIT. During this state, protection depends on the regular ingestion of the food allergen; when dosing is interrupted or discontinued, the protective effect may be lost or significantly decreased. By tracking ex vivo changes in peripheral peanut-reactive T cells in particpants during OIT, the authors' group recently observed a strong correlation between decrease of peanut-specific TH2 cells and achievement of peanut desensitization.[52] Interestingly, remaining allergen-specific T-cell subtypes, which share similar features with those seen in nonallergic individuals, remain unchanged. Similarly, a mechanistic study using single-cell sorting and transcriptional profiling of individual T cells collected throughout OIT showed that induction of anergic T cells along with decreased allergen-specific TH2 cells accompanied oral desensitization.[65]

The ultimate goal of OIT is to restore permanent oral tolerance, which is established when food may be ingested without allergic symptoms, despite prolonged periods of avoidance. A phase 1 peanut-OIT study by Syed and colleagues[66] targeted such identification of specific immune mechanisms associated with a tolerant clinical phenotype. Although they observed that serum IgE or IgG4 level along with basophil activation did not statistically differentiate between clinical "immune tolerance" and "immune desensitization," epigenetic changes in antigen-induced Treg cells were shown to be predictive of long-lasting clinical benefit after the withdrawal of OIT. In murine experimental models of food allergy, it has been shown that cow's milk OIT induced LP pTreg cells that controlled the allergic reaction through the production of IL-10 and TGF-β.[67] Interestingly, in their model, the adoptive transfer of FoxP3+ Treg resulted in pronounced disease exacerbation, thus confirming that Treg cells have an essential role in resolving food allergy.[33] One possible mechanism to explain and integrate all these results into a cohesive schema is that restoration of permanent oral tolerance is a stepwise process that likely involves the initial anergy and deletion of allergen-specific TH2 cells (desensitization state) followed by the development of allergen-specific T cells with stable regulatory properties at later stages (tolerance state).[68] However, local immune mechanisms associated with OIT remain to be further investigated, most particularly with respect to cells involved in allergen uptake at the administration site.

SUMMARY

Oral tolerance to dietary antigens and commensal bacteria is crucial to prevent the development of food allergies, celiac disease, and autoimmune diseases. The oral route of administration takes advantage of the unique set of immune cells and pathways involved in the induction of oral tolerance. Early microbial colonization and exposure to solid food plays an important role in promoting natural oral tolerance. OIT is thought to initiate desensitization through interaction of an allergen with mucosal DCs that initiate downstream immune system modulation through Tregs and effector T cells. Future in-depth understanding of the process involved in the restoration of oral tolerance through OIT will likely contribute to a more effective treatment of disease.

REFERENCES

1. Goubier A, Dubois B, Gheit H, et al. Plasmacytoid dendritic cells mediate oral tolerance. Immunity 2008;29:464–75.

45. Myles IA. Fast food fever: reviewing the impacts of the Western diet on immunity. Nutr J 2014;13:61.
46. Tan J, McKenzie C, Vuillermin PJ, et al. Dietary fiber and bacterial SCFA enhance oral tolerance and protect against food allergy through diverse cellular pathways. Cell Rep 2016;15:2809–24.
47. Chewning JH, Weaver CT. Development and survival of Th17 cells within the intestines: the influence of microbiome- and diet-derived signals. J Immunol 2014; 193:4769–77.
48. Clayburgh DR, Musch MW, Leitges M, et al. Coordinated epithelial NHE3 inhibition and barrier dysfunction are required for TNF-mediated diarrhea in vivo. J Clin Invest 2006;116:2682–94.
49. Venkataraman D, Soto-Ramirez N, Kurukulaaratchy RJ, et al. Filaggrin loss-of-function mutations are associated with food allergy in childhood and adolescence. J Allergy Clin Immunol 2014;134:876–82.e4.
50. Laffont S, Siddiqui KR, Powrie F. Intestinal inflammation abrogates the tolerogenic properties of MLN CD103+ dendritic cells. Eur J Immunol 2010;40:1877–83.
51. Bulek K, Swaidani S, Aronica M, et al. Epithelium: the interplay between innate and Th2 immunity. Immunol Cell Biol 2010;88:257–68.
52. Wambre E, Bajzik V, DeLong JH, et al. A phenotypically and functionally distinct human TH2 cell subpopulation is associated with allergic disorders. Sci Transl Med 2017;9(401):1–10.
53. Mitson-Salazar A, Yin Y, Wansley DL, et al. Hematopoietic prostaglandin D synthase defines a proeosinophilic pathogenic effector human T(H)2 cell subpopulation with enhanced function. J Allergy Clin Immunol 2016;137:907–18.e9.
54. Lam EP, Kariyawasam HH, Rana BM, et al. IL-25/IL-33-responsive TH2 cells characterize nasal polyps with a default TH17 signature in nasal mucosa. J Allergy Clin Immunol 2016;137:1514–24.
55. Van Dyken SJ, Nussbaum JC, Lee J, et al. A tissue checkpoint regulates type 2 immunity. Nat Immunol 2016;17:1381–7.
56. Endo Y, Hirahara K, Yagi R, et al. Pathogenic memory type Th2 cells in allergic inflammation. Trends Immunology 2014;35:69–78.
57. von Moltke J, Ji M, Liang HE, et al. Tuft-cell-derived IL-25 regulates an intestinal ILC2-epithelial response circuit. Nature 2016;529:221–5.
58. Lee JB, Chen CY, Liu B, et al. IL-25 and CD4(+) TH2 cells enhance type 2 innate lymphoid cell-derived IL-13 production, which promotes IgE-mediated experimental food allergy. J Allergy Clin Immunol 2016;137:1216–25.e5.
59. Mathias CB, Hobson SA, Garcia-Lloret M, et al. IgE-mediated systemic anaphylaxis and impaired tolerance to food antigens in mice with enhanced IL-4 receptor signaling. J Allergy Clin Immunol 2011;127:795–805.e1-8.
60. Schofield A. A case of egg poisoning. Lancet 1908;171:716.
61. Konieczna P, Ferstl R, Ziegler M, et al. Immunomodulation by Bifidobacterium infantis 35624 in the murine lamina propria requires retinoic acid-dependent and independent mechanisms. PLoS One 2013;8:e62617.
62. Perezabad L, Reche M, Valbuena T, et al. Oral food desensitization in children with IgE-mediated cow's milk allergy: immunological changes underlying desensitization. Allergy Asthma Immunol Res 2017;9:35–42.
63. Berin MC, Mayer L. Can we produce true tolerance in patients with food allergy? J Allergy Clin Immunol 2013;131:14–22.
64. Shreffler WG, Wanich N, Moloney M, et al. Association of allergen-specific regulatory T cells with the onset of clinical tolerance to milk protein. J Allergy Clin Immunol 2009;123:43–52.e7.

65. Ryan JF, Hovde R, Glanville J, et al. Successful immunotherapy induces previously unidentified allergen-specific CD4+ T-cell subsets. Proc Natl Acad Sci United States America 2016;113:E1286–95.
66. Syed A, Garcia MA, Lyu SC, et al. Peanut oral immunotherapy results in increased antigen-induced regulatory T-cell function and hypomethylation of forkhead box protein 3 (FOXP3). J Allergy Clin Immunol 2014;133:500–10.
67. Smaldini PL, Orsini Delgado ML, Fossati CA, et al. Orally-induced intestinal CD4+ CD25+ FoxP3+ Treg controlled undesired responses towards oral antigens and effectively dampened food allergic reactions. PLoS One 2015;10: e0141116.
68. Wambre E. Effect of allergen-specific immunotherapy on CD4+ T cells. Curr Opin Allergy Clin Immunol 2015;15:581–7.

Diagnosis of Food Allergy

Malika Gupta, MD[a], Amanda Cox, MD[b],
Anna Nowak-Węgrzyn, MD, PhD[b], Julie Wang, MD[b],*

KEYWORDS

- Diagnosis • Food allergy • Molecular allergen analysis • Serum-specific IgE
- Skin prick test • Epitope binding • Basophil activation test
- Component-resolved diagnostic testing

KEY POINTS

- Differentiating between clinical allergy and sensitization is challenging but important to prevent overdiagnosis of food allergy.
- Double-blind placebo controlled food-challenges remain the gold standard for the diagnosis of food allergy, although their utility remains limited to research studies. In clinical settings, open oral food challenges are usually considered sufficient.
- Standard food allergy diagnosis involves the use of skin prick tests, allergen-specific immunoglobulin E, and oral food challenges. Molecular allergen analysis is a promising new technique and has increased specificity of testing for peanut and hazelnut allergies, with attention now shifting to other food allergens. Basophil activation tests and epitope binding are actively used in research and may have clinical applications for diagnosis of food allergy in the future.

INTRODUCTION

Food allergy (FA) is defined as "an adverse health effect arising from a specific immune response that occurs reproducibly on exposure to a given food."[1] FA prevalence increased by almost 50% over the past 2 decades in countries with a Western lifestyle.[2] FA is estimated to affect 6% to 8% of the children in the United States and approximately 3% to 4% of the adults.[3] This has led to an increased focus on all aspects of FA, from prevention to treatment.

Diagnosis of FA is challenging, with pitfalls associated with most testing methods. Despite several advances, a double-blind, placebo-controlled food challenge (DBPCFC) remains the gold standard for FA diagnosis. Correctly identifying FA is

Disclosure Statement: The authors have no relevant financial disclosures or conflicts of interests.
[a] Division of Allergy & Immunology, Department of Internal Medicine, University of Michigan, 24 Frank Lloyd Wright Drive, Suite H-2100, Ann Arbor, MI 48106, USA; [b] Department of Pediatrics, Icahn School of Medicine at Mount Sinai, Jaffe Food Allergy Institute, One Gustave Levy Place, Box 1198, New York, NY 10029, USA
* Corresponding author.
E-mail address: Julie.Wang@mssm.edu

Immunol Allergy Clin N Am 38 (2018) 39–52
https://doi.org/10.1016/j.iac.2017.09.004
0889-8561/18/© 2017 Elsevier Inc. All rights reserved.

important, not only to prevent reactions but also to avoid unnecessary dietary restrictions that negatively affect growth.[4,5]

This article describes the diagnostic methods for immunoglobulin E (IgE)-mediated FA with a particular focus on molecular allergen analysis (MAA) and basophil activation testing (BAT). This article does not include evaluation of non–IgE-mediated food-allergies, which involve different diagnostic approaches.

CLINICAL HISTORY

As with any disease, a detailed history is important and guides further testing:

- A description of typical symptoms of IgE-mediated allergy (described in **Table 1**), timing of symptoms in relation to food ingestion (usually minutes to 1–2 hours), reproducibility of symptoms with subsequent food ingestion, form (eg, raw vs cooked), and amount of food ingested, are all relevant in FA diagnosis.
- It is important to rule out conditions that mimic FA (**Box 1**).
- Certain populations are at higher risk of FA: those with eczema, asthma, allergic rhinitis, other FA, and a family history of atopic disease (AD).[6]
- Associated cofactors, including acute febrile illness, asthma exacerbation, exercise, alcohol ingestion, drugs increasing gastric pH, and nonsteroidal antiinflammatory drugs, can worsen the severity of an allergic reaction and should be assessed.[7]
- Knowledge of cross-reactivity within food protein families should guide further tests to exclude allergy to related foods if they have not yet been ingested. This should be done cautiously because testing for all homologous proteins can result in elimination of foods that demonstrate sensitization but may not result in allergic reactions.[8] **Fig. 1** summarizes the approximate rate of cross-reactivity between different foods.[8] Decisions regarding testing should be based on likelihood of allergy and the nutritional and social importance of the food.

STANDARD TESTING

In addition to a detailed clinical history, several diagnostic tests can be considered in the evaluation of FA.

Table 1 System-based symptoms encountered in acute immunoglobulin E–mediated food reactions	
System Involved	Symptoms (Usual Onset Within Minutes to 1–2 h Following Food Ingestion)
Cutaneous	Pruritus, flushing, urticaria, angioedema, flare of chronic eczematous rash
Ocular	Pruritus, conjunctival erythema, tearing, periorbital edema
Respiratory tract	Nasal congestion, pruritus, sneezing, laryngeal edema and hoarseness, cough, wheeze, chest tightness, dyspnea, cyanosis
Gastrointestinal	Nausea; emesis; crampy abdominal pain; oral pruritus; tongue, lip, palate, or pharyngeal angioedema
Cardiovascular	Tachycardia, bradycardia, hypotension, cardiac arrest, dizziness
Neurologic	Sense of impending doom, syncope, dizziness

Adapted from Sampson HA, Aceves S, Bock SA, et al. Food allergy: a practice parameter update-2014. J Allergy Clin Immunol 2014;134(5):1025.e41; with permission.

Box 1
Differential diagnosis for food allergy

- Allergic reactions to drugs, venom, inhalants
- Food intolerance (eg, lactose intolerance)
- Toxic reactions or food poisoning (eg, scombroid fish toxin, poisoning due to *Escherichia coli*)
- Pharmacologic reactions (eg, to caffeine, theobromine, alcohol)
- Auriculotemporal syndrome (Frey syndrome)
- Gustatory rhinitis caused by spicy foods
- Panic, anorexia nervosa

Data from Sampson HA, Aceves S, Bock SA, et al. Food allergy: a practice parameter update-2014. J Allergy Clin Immunol 2014;134(5):1025.e42.

The diagnostic pathway commonly begins with a skin prick test (SPT) for the suspected allergen with or without a serum-specific IgE (ssIgE). Both tests detect antigen-specific IgE (asIgE). The presence of asIgE is called sensitization and alone does not confirm FA because asIgE can be present in the absence of clinical allergy.[1] Therefore, these tests must be interpreted in the context of clinical history. A larger SPT diameter or a higher ssIgE correspond to a higher likelihood of clinical reaction[7,9] but do not predict the severity of a reaction. The advent of MAA has made it possible to identify sensitization to allergens predicting systemic reactions.

SKIN PRICK TESTING

During SPT procedure, the skin surface is pricked with allergen to measure the asIgE bound to cutaneous mast cells.[7] SPT results in a wheal and flare response, which is measured within 15 minutes.[10] SPT has limited utility in patients with dermatographism or who are taking systemic antihistamines.[1] Wheal sizes vary with age, body site used for testing (usually greater on back compared with forearms), device used, the potency and commercial extract manufacturer, or if fresh food is used. The negative predictive value (NPV) of SPT is greater than 90%, making it a useful test for excluding FA in the absence of a convincing clinical history.[7] This is especially true for the major allergens for which commercial skin test extracts are available.[11] False-negative SPT may occur if the commercial extracts are not standardized and lack the allergen in sufficient quantities.[12] This is particularly true for fruits and vegetables in which the antigens are destroyed during the manufacturing process.[12] In these cases, prick-prick testing with the fresh food may be used.[7]

The positive predictive value (PPV) of SPT depends on the patient's age and the food allergen,[7] and can differ with the SPT method used and presence of atopy. The 95% PPV values have been established for only a few major food allergens (summarized in **Table 2**). In general, a larger SPT correlates with an increased likelihood of reaction.[7]

SPT should be performed by a trained personnel in a facility capable of managing anaphylaxis, which can rarely be triggered by SPT. Intradermal skin testing is not recommended in FA diagnosis because it can provoke anaphylaxis and is associated with high rates of false-positive results.[7]

SERUM FOOD ALLERGEN–SPECIFIC IMMUNOGLOBULIN E

Extract-based in vitro testing for allergen-specific IgE in serum (ssIgE) is another diagnostic tool. Physicians can send ssIgE from the office and it can be used in patients

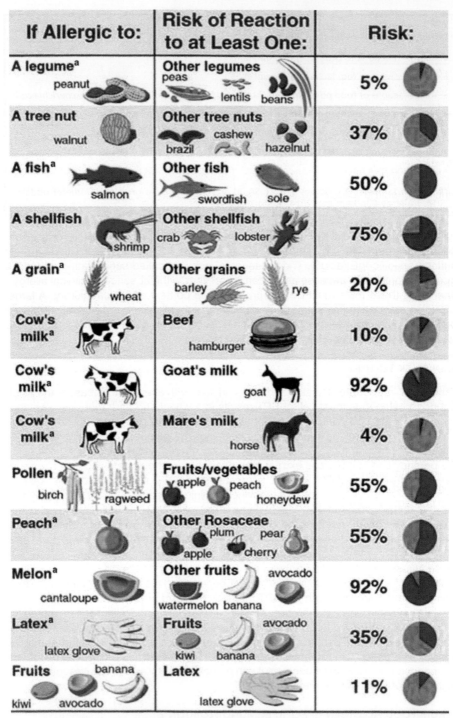

Fig. 1. Cross-reactive foods.[a] Data derived from studies with DBPCFCs. (*From* Sicherer SH. Clinical implications of cross-reactive food allergens. J Allergy Clin Immunol 2001;108(6):885; with permission.)

Table 2
Predictive values for skin prick testing in positive or negative oral food challenges

Food	95% Positive (mm)[a]	50% Negative (mm)[b]
Egg white	≥7	≤3
Cow's milk	≥8	—
Peanut	≥8	≤3

[a] Mean wheal diameters above which 95% of the challenges are expected to be positive (failed).
[b] Mean wheal diameters under which 50% of the challenges are expected to be negative (passed).
Adapted from Sampson HA, Aceves S, Bock SA, et al. Food allergy: a practice parameter update-2014. J Allergy Clin Immunol 2014;134(5):1025.e42; with permission.

who are unable to cooperate with skin testing, those with extensive skin disease, or those unable to discontinue oral antihistamines.

Serum allergen-specific IgE has high sensitivity but low specificity for FA.[13] A detectable ssIgE by itself is not diagnostic of FA, but increasing ssIgE levels correlate with increased likelihood of a true allergy.[9] Of note, in 10% to 25% of cases, reactions can occur with undetectable ssIgE.[14] This may be explained by insufficient sensitivity of the immunoassay and/or loss of minor allergens during extract preparation for the immunoassay.

Predictive values of clinical reactivity have been established for several foods (summarized in **Table 3**). When ssIgE levels are greater than or equal to 95% PPV, FA is likely. If ssIgE levels are less than or equal to 50% PPV, a physician-supervised oral food challenge (OFC) can be considered to exclude FA. These cutoff values have been established based on ImmunoCAP (ThermoFisher, Waltham, Massachusetts, USA) and are not comparable to the levels measured by other immunoassays.[15] The cutoff values differ with age because lower ssIgE antibody levels have higher PPV in infants and younger children.[7] They are also affected by the prior history of reactions, which is associated with a higher pretest probability.[7]

Few studies have suggested interpreting allergen-ssIgE in the context of the total IgE for improved accuracy.[16,17] Further studies are needed before this method can be used clinically. Although no single factor is thought to be an absolute predictor by itself, using a combination of factors might increase the accuracy of predictive models. DunnGalvin and colleagues[18] developed predictive models for peanut, milk, and egg using 6 clinical

Table 3
Predictive values for food allergen–specific immunoglobulin E for children

Allergen	≥95% Predictive Level (kUA/L)	PPV
Egg	7	98
Infants ≤2 y	2	95
Cow milk	15	95
Infants ≤2 y	5	95
Peanut	14	100
Fish	20	100
Tree nuts	15	≈ 95
Soybean	30	73
Wheat	26	74

Adapted from Sampson HA. Update on food allergy. J Allergy Clin Immunol 2004;113(5):812 [quiz: 820]; with permission.

factors: SPT, ssIgE, total IgE minus ssIgE, symptoms, sex, and age. The sensitivity and specificity of the Cork-Southampton algorithm incorporating these 6 variables was higher than using SPT, or ssIgE, or a combination of SPT and ssIgE. Age tends to be an important predictor in these models, whereas time since the last reaction seems to be less important.[18] Also, the relative importance of an individual factor varies by food.[18]

In infants, ssIgE might be more sensitive than SPT. In the Learning Early About Peanut Allergy (LEAP) study, which enrolled infants in the 4 to 11 months age group, almost 28% of infants with negative skin tests had detectable peanut-ssIgE.[19] Race also affects the PPV of ssIgE levels. Black race is more commonly associated with higher ssIgE levels[19,20] but less clinical reactivity. In the LEAP study, it was noted that higher peanut ssIgE levels in the black subjects were often associated with negative SPT, and no clinical reactivity compared with other races. Thus, SPT was assumed to be a more accurate predictor in black subjects.[19,21]

The FA guidelines suggest combining SPT and ssIgE to increase the PPV and NPV for the diagnosis of FA.[1]

Other uses of ssIgE include periodic monitoring of the longitudinal trend to determine the resolution of FA.[14,22] Regarding egg and milk, a 50% decrease in ssIgE over 12 months is more likely predictive of resolution of allergy compared with a slower decrease over a long period of time.[22]

Children with higher peak lifetime ssIgE (generally above 50 kilounits of allergen-specific IgE per liter [kUA/L]) are more likely to have persistent cow's milk, egg, soy, and wheat allergy.[23]

The Consortium for Food Allergy Research developed a Web-based calculator to counsel families about the prognosis of milk allergy in children younger than 15 months (www.cofargroup.org). The calculator is based on milk-ssIgE, SPT, and severity of AD, which are most predictive of milk allergy resolution (**Fig. 2**).[24] A prognostic calculator for egg allergy is also available.[25]

MOLECULAR ALLERGEN ANALYSIS

MAA (aka component-resolved diagnostic testing) augments the accuracy of conventional testing.[26] Conventional ssIgE measures IgE to the whole food extract, which contains both allergenic and nonallergic components.[27] MAA, on the other hand, identifies IgE bound to specific protein antigens in a food.[27]

MAA can separate the clinically relevant from the irrelevant IgE with prognostic benefit.[27] This is most helpful either when 1 main isoform of the protein is associated with the allergic reaction or when the allergen is degraded easily by heat or digestion. Proteins that are resistant to heat or digestion are more likely to cause systemic reactions. For instance, ovomucoid is a heat-resistant egg white protein. Individuals who are predominantly sensitized to ovomucoid are less likely to tolerate baked egg products[28] and MAA helps identify this phenotype.

MAA can also be applied to evaluating sensitization to foods that share homologous proteins with aeroallergens.[26] Patients primarily sensitized to the hazelnut Cor a 1, which is a homolog of Bet v 1, are more likely to experience mild oral or no symptoms compared with patients sensitized to the storage seed proteins (Cor a 9, Cor a 14) who are more likely to experience systemic symptoms.[29]

The ratio of component-specific IgE to total IgE does not improve the predictive ability of MAA, high total IgE levels lower the probability of positive challenges at a given Ara h2 and Cor A 14 for peanut and hazelnut, respectively.[30]

Two commercial immunoassays measure IgE to individual food allergens. Fluorescent enzyme immunoassay (ImmunoCAP) uses purified native or recombinant

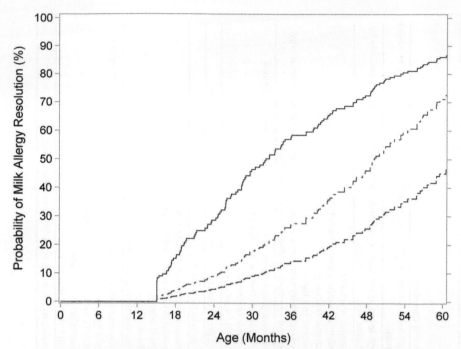

Fig. 2. Predicting the natural history of resolution of milk allergy. Red curve represents a patient with milk ssIgE of 20 kUA/L, milk SPT mean of 7 mm, and moderate-to-severe AD.
Green curve represents a patient with milk ssIgE of 20 kUA/L, milk SPT mean of 7 mm,
and mild to no AD. Blue curve represents a patient with milk ssIgE of 2 kUA/L, milk SPT
mean of 4 mm, and mild to no AD. (*From* Wood RA, Sicherer SH, Vickery BP, et al. The natural history of milk allergy in an observational cohort. J Allergy Clin Immunol
2013;131(3):811; with permission.)

proteins and provides quantitative results expressed as kUA/L. A microarray-based
immunoassay (ImmunoCAP ISAC) measures specific IgE to greater than 100 allergens
simultaneously.[31] The results obtained from ISAC are semiquantitative and are
expressed in ISAC standardized units (ISUs).[31] Notably, because ISAC covers a
wide spectrum of food allergens, this type of testing has the potential of overdiagnos-
ing food allergies by detecting sensitization to foods that may not be clinically relevant.

Peanut-MAA is best-studied and most often used in practice. Although Ara h 1, 2,
and 3 have all been associated with systemic peanut allergy; Ara h 2 has is the best
predictor of peanut allergy with sensitivity approaching 100% and specificity
approaching 96.1% in 1 study.[32] In contrast, monosensitization to Ara h 8 (a homo-
logue of the labile birch protein Bet v 1) is usually associated with mild oral to no symptoms. These patients should undergo physician-supervised OFCs because they are
likely to tolerate peanut. Of note, Ara h 6 is also associated with systemic reactions
but is only available with ISAC.[33] Clinically important major food allergens are summarized in **Table 4**.

BASOPHIL ACTIVATION TEST

An allergic reaction is provoked when allergen crosslinks FcεRI-bound surface membrane IgE on basophils and mast cells, which then degranulate to release histamine

Table 4
Clinically important major food allergens

Food	Major Allergen	Clinical Correlation
Cow's milk[28]	Bos d 8 (casein)	High levels of casein-IgE indicate higher likelihood of reactivity to baked milk
Egg[28]	Gal d 1 (ovomucoid)	High levels of ovomucoid-IgE indicate higher likelihood of reactivity to baked egg
Peanut[34]	Ara h 1	Systemic reactivity
	Ara h 2	Systemic reactivity (best predictor)
	Ara h 3	Systemic reactivity
	Ara h 6	Systemic reactivity
	Ara h 8	Cross-reactivity with Bet v 1 (usually tolerant or with mild oral allergy)
	Ara h 9	Systemic reactivity in Mediterranean regions[35]
Hazelnut[29]	Cor a 1	Cross-reacts with Bet v 1; no correlation with systemic reactions
	Cor a 8	Systemic reactivity in Mediterranean regions[36]
	Cor a 9	Systemic reactions
	Cor a 14	Systemic reactions
Cashew[37]	Ana o 3	Best predictor of systemic allergy to cashew and pistachio
Walnut[38]	Jug r 1	Anaphylactic reactions
Wheat[39–41]	Tri a 14	Clinical reactivity in Mediterranean regions
	Tri a 19 (Omega 5-gliadin)	Correlates with severe wheat allergy, WDEIA
	Tri a 20	Wheat allergy
	Tri a 21	Wheat allergy
	Tri a 36	Cross-reactivity with other cereal grains
Soy[42]	Gly m 4	Cross-reactivity with Bet v 1, correlates with milder symptoms or oral allergy symptoms
	Gly m 5	Systemic symptoms in the absence of Gly m 5 and 6
	Gly m 6	Anaphylactic reactions
		Anaphylactic reactions
Beef, lamb, pork meat[43]	Galactose-alpha-1,3-galactose (alpha-gal)	Predicts delayed reactions to mammalian meat

Abbreviation: WDEIA, wheat-dependent exercise-induced anaphylaxis.

and other mediators. BAT mimics an allergic reaction and reflects a functional response rather than sensitization.[44] Flow cytometry detects surface activation markers, usually CD63 and CD203c, on the allergen-stimulated basophils.[44] BAT should ideally be able to distinguish between clinically allergic and sensitized-but-tolerant individuals.[45] BAT may also predict anaphylaxis.[46]

Crude allergen extracts and purified or recombinant allergens can be used to stimulate basophils for BAT.[47] BAT results may be reported as basophil reactivity or basophil sensitivity. Basophil reactivity is reported as the maximum proportion (CD-max) of activated basophils measured at any concentration of stimulating allergen. Basophil sensitivity (EC50 or CDsens) is the smallest effective allergen concentration causing 50% of maximal basophil activation.[44] An area under the dose-responsive curve, which provides a measurement of both basophil reactivity and sensitivity, may also be measured.[44]

BAT has high sensitivity and specificity for diagnosis of peanut, hazelnut, egg, milk, and wheat allergies, as well as for pollen-food syndrome to apple, hazelnut, celery, and carrot.[45]

BAT assays generally have comparable sensitivity to SPT and ssIgE but improved specificity as a diagnostic test for FA. In cases in which SPT and ssIgE provide equivocal or inconclusive results, BAT may be useful as an intermediate step before proceeding with an OFC to confirm tolerance or FA.

BAT differentiates between FA phenotypes. For example, milk-specific basophil reactivity is greater in baked milk–reactive children compared with baked milk–tolerant but nonheated milk–reactive children.[48] BAT results also correlate with DBPCFC severity scores in a study of 12- to 45-year-olds with peanut, tree nut, fish, shrimp, and sesame allergy.[46]

BAT may be useful in evaluating for the resolution of food allergies, such as milk,[49] wheat,[50] and egg,[51] which are often outgrown, and for helping determine when these may be safely reintroduced into a child's diet. Decreased basophil sensitivity and reactivity have been observed for patients with clinical response (desensitization) to sublingual and oral immunotherapy for peanut,[52] cow's milk,[53] and egg.[54] BAT may eventually be used to assess the development of clinical tolerance and response to immune-modulating therapies for FA.

BAT remains a research modality and is not likely to be used as a stand-alone test for the diagnosis of FA. Additional studies are needed to standardize the laboratory assay methods and validate BAT values for different food allergens and for different populations, as well as for assessing the utility of BAT for monitoring natural resolution of FA and clinical response to emerging therapies for FA. BAT results may eventually be considered in combination with other diagnostic tests, and may improve the safety of and reduce the number of OFCs.

EPITOPE ANALYSIS

Conventional serologic and MAA testing evaluate ssIgE responses to whole proteins, whereas epitope mapping allows for analysis of IgE-binding to specific segments of allergenic proteins (epitopes). Immunodominant epitopes are those that bind the most food-specific IgE and are recognized by most patients with clinical FA. IgE-binding epitopes may be sequential or conformational. Sequential epitopes are composed of a linear sequence of neighboring amino acids in a protein. Conformational epitopes include amino acids that are not sequential and are only brought together when a protein is in its tertiary (or folded) conformation.

Conformational epitopes are more susceptible to degradation by heating and enzymatic digestion, and thus may be less allergenic than linear epitopes.[28] Patients with

IgE recognizing sequential epitopes of ovalbumin and ovomucoid have more persistent egg allergy than those who primarily bind conformational epitopes.[55]

Using protein microarray, IgE-binding to multiple short linear allergen peptides in a food allergen can also be analyzed.[56] This epitope analysis has been applied for milk, egg, and peanut. For milk allergy, patients with IgE to multiple linear allergenic epitopes in beta-lactoglobulin may have persistent cow's milk allergy compared with those who only recognize conformational epitopes on alpha-lactalbumin.[57] IgE binding to a higher number of epitopes with greater affinity may also be predictive of more severe allergic reactions, reactivity to baked milk, and more persistent milk allergy.[58] Similarly, higher epitope diversity corresponds to clinical sensitivity and severity of peanut allergy.[59]

Although epitope analysis is still primarily a research modality, it may prove to be an additional tool for diagnosing symptomatic FA, differentiating among various phenotypes, and determining prognosis.

ORAL FOOD CHALLENGE

A DBPCFC is the gold standard for FA diagnosis, although single-blind and open (unblinded) OFCs, despite being more subject to bias and having more frequent false-positive results, are more practical in most clinical settings.[60]

The decision to conduct an OFC should be guided by a patient's clinical history, ssIgE, and/or SPT.[60] Additional diagnostic tests, once standardized, may eventually also factor into the decision to perform an OFC. An OFC should not be considered if history and/or testing are convincing that the food will provoke an acute allergic reaction. An OFC may be performed if the patient history is uncertain, or if diagnostic testing is negative, inconclusive, or below threshold levels predictive of clinical reactivity.[7]

An OFC is also warranted if clinical history or diagnostic testing indicates that FA may have resolved. The social and nutritional benefits of adding the challenge food to a patient's diet should be taken into consideration. The risks, including the potential for provoking a severe allergic reaction, and emotional consequences of not tolerating the food, should be considered carefully when deciding to perform an OFC.

The OFC should be performed in a facility where medical personnel are trained, fully equipped, and prepared to treat anaphylaxis.[60]

During an OFC, the food should be given gradually in incremental doses to minimize the risk of anaphylaxis and help identify the lowest provoking dose.[60] Various forms and preparations of foods may be used, as well as different starting and total doses. Baking decreases the allergenicity of milk and egg, and may not provoke a reaction in individuals allergic to fresh or raw forms of milk and egg.[28] Allergenicity of beef, seafood, fruits, and vegetables can also be affected by preparation and cooking methods.[28] For blinded challenges, the food needs to be mixed with an appropriate vehicle that masks its taste, smell, and texture.[60] A placebo-food may also be incorporated into the challenge. Published protocols differ with regard to number and timing of dosing intervals, as well as observation periods; however, most OFCs are generally performed over several hours.[60]

OFC should be discontinued if symptoms develop and treatment rendered immediately. In negative OFC (absent allergic symptoms), the patient may subsequently introduce the challenged food into their diet at home and they should be instructed to ingest the food regularly to maintain tolerance. Patients should be instructed to continue avoidance of any food that provokes an allergic reaction during OFC. Education and guidance should be provided to families for successful and safe avoidance of food allergens (https://web.emmes.com/study/cofar/EducationProgram.htm).

Special considerations need to be taken when conducting OFCs in infants. With current guidelines recommending early introduction of peanut to infants at high risk for developing peanut allergy, there will likely be an increased demand for peanut-OFCs for infants 4 to 11 months of age who have early onset AD (severe eczema and/or egg allergy).[19] A workgroup report from the Adverse Reactions to Foods Committee of the American Academy of Allergy, Asthma, and Immunology provides specific infant peanut-OFC guidance, taking into consideration infant developmental stages and age-appropriate forms, textures, and amounts of peanut that may be offered.[61]

UNPROVEN METHODS

Allergen specific-IgG measurement, applied kinesiology, cytotoxicity assays, and gastric juice analysis are not recommended in the diagnosis of FA.[7] These are discussed (See Catherine Hammond and Jay A. Lieberman's article, "Unproven Diagnostic Tests for Food Allergy," in this issue for further details).

SUMMARY

FA is rapidly evolving in the wake of increased prevalence and increased awareness among clinicians and parents alike. Promising new diagnostic methods, such as MAA, BAT, and epitope mapping, are under active investigation. Although early data are encouraging, more robust studies must be performed before these tests can be used clinically.

Standard testing for FA involves SPT and ssIgE. These tests are sensitive but not specific and must be interpreted with caution. Although some highly predictive SPT and ssIgE threshold levels have been determined for milk, egg, and peanut allergies, these levels are not well described for most other allergens. Attention is now focused on MAA, which will likely add to the specificity of FA diagnosis. The future of FA diagnosis perhaps lies in the use of multiple diagnostic parameters, along with clinical history to increase accuracy and to minimize dependence on OFCs.

REFERENCES

1. Boyce JA, Assa'ad A, Burks AW, et al. Guidelines for the diagnosis and management of food allergy in the United States: report of the NIAID-sponsored expert panel. J Allergy Clin Immunol 2010;126(6 Suppl):S1–58.
2. Jackson KD, Howie LD, Akinbami LJ. Trends in allergic conditions among children: United States, 1997-2011. NCHS Data Brief 2013;(121):1–8.
3. Gupta RS, Springston EE, Warrier MR, et al. The prevalence, severity, and distribution of childhood food allergy in the United States. Pediatrics 2011;128(1):e9–17.
4. Mehta H, Groetch M, Wang J. Growth and nutritional concerns in children with food allergy. Curr Opin Allergy Clin Immunol 2013;13(3):275–9.
5. Robbins KA, Guerrerio AL, Hauck SA, et al. Growth and nutrition in children with food allergy requiring amino acid-based nutritional formulas. J Allergy Clin Immunol 2014;134(6):1463–6.e5.
6. Spergel JM, Paller AS. Atopic dermatitis and the atopic march. J Allergy Clin Immunol 2003;112(6 Suppl):S118–27.
7. Sampson HA, Aceves S, Bock SA, et al. Food allergy: a practice parameter update-2014. J Allergy Clin Immunol 2014;134(5):1016–25.e43.
8. Sicherer SH. Clinical implications of cross-reactive food allergens. J Allergy Clin Immunol 2001;108(6):881–90.

9. Perry TT, Matsui EC, Kay Conover-Walker M, et al. The relationship of allergen-specific IgE levels and oral food challenge outcome. J Allergy Clin Immunol 2004;114(1):144–9.

10. Khan FM, Ueno-Yamanouchi A, Serushago B, et al. Basophil activation test compared to skin prick test and fluorescence enzyme immunoassay for aeroallergen-specific Immunoglobulin-E. Allergy Asthma Clin Immunol 2012; 8(1):1.

11. Chokshi NY, Sicherer SH. Interpreting IgE sensitization tests in food allergy. Expert Rev Clin Immunol 2016;12(4):389–403.

12. Nowak-Wegrzyn A, Burks W, Sampson HA. Chapter 81: reactions to foods. In: Middleton E, Franklin Adkinson N, Busse WW, et al, editors. Middleton's allergy: principles and practice, vol. 2, 8th edition. Philadelphia: W B Saunders; 2014. p. 1237–59.

13. Soares-Weiser K, Takwoingi Y, Panesar SS, et al. The diagnosis of food allergy: a systematic review and meta-analysis. Allergy 2014;69(1):76–86.

14. Sampson HA. Utility of food-specific IgE concentrations in predicting symptomatic food allergy. J Allergy Clin Immunol 2001;107(5):891–6.

15. Wang J, Godbold JH, Sampson HA. Correlation of serum allergy (IgE) tests performed by different assay systems. J Allergy Clin Immunol 2008;121(5):1219–24.

16. Federly TJ, Jones BL, Dai H, et al. Interpretation of food specific immunoglobulin E levels in the context of total IgE. Ann Allergy Asthma Immunol 2013;111(1): 20–4.

17. Gupta RS, Lau CH, Hamilton RG, et al. Predicting outcomes of oral food challenges by using the allergen-specific IgE-total IgE ratio. J Allergy Clin Immunol Pract 2014;2(3):300–5.

18. DunnGalvin A, Daly D, Cullinane C, et al. Highly accurate prediction of food challenge outcome using routinely available clinical data. J Allergy Clin Immunol 2011;127(3):633–9.e1-3.

19. Du Toit G, Roberts G, Sayre PH, et al. Randomized trial of peanut consumption in infants at risk for peanut allergy. N Engl J Med 2015;372(9):803–13.

20. Maloney JM, Nowak-Wegrzyn A, Wang J. Children in the inner city of New York have high rates of food allergy and IgE sensitization to common foods. J Allergy Clin Immunol 2011;128(1):214–5.

21. Du Toit G, Roberts G, Sayre PH, et al. Identifying infants at high risk of peanut allergy: the Learning Early About Peanut Allergy (LEAP) screening study. J Allergy Clin Immunol 2013;131(1):135–43.e1-12.

22. Shek LP, Soderstrom L, Ahlstedt S, et al. Determination of food specific IgE levels over time can predict the development of tolerance in cow's milk and hen's egg allergy. J Allergy Clin Immunol 2004;114(2):387–91.

23. Savage J, Sicherer S, Wood R. The natural history of food allergy. J Allergy Clin Immunol Pract 2016;4(2):196–203 [quiz: 204].

24. Wood RA, Sicherer SH, Vickery BP, et al. The natural history of milk allergy in an observational cohort. J Allergy Clin Immunol 2013;131(3):805–12.

25. Sicherer SH, Wood RA, Vickery BP, et al. The natural history of egg allergy in an observational cohort. J Allergy Clin Immunol 2014;133(2):492–9.

26. Matricardi PM, Kleine-Tebbe J, Hoffmann HJ, et al. EAACI molecular allergology user's guide. Pediatr Allergy Immunol 2016;27(Suppl 23):1–250.

27. Treudler R, Simon JC. Overview of component resolved diagnostics. Curr Allergy Asthma Rep 2013;13(1):110–7.

28. Nowak-Wegrzyn A, Fiocchi A. Rare, medium, or well done? The effect of heating and food matrix on food protein allergenicity. Curr Opin Allergy Clin Immunol 2009;9(3):234–7.

29. Kattan JD, Sicherer SH, Sampson HA. Clinical reactivity to hazelnut may be better identified by component testing than traditional testing methods. J Allergy Clin Immunol Prac 2014;2(5):633–4.e1.

30. Grabenhenrich L, Lange L, Hartl M, et al. The component-specific to total IgE ratios do not improve peanut and hazelnut allergy diagnoses. J Allergy Clin Immunol 2016;137(6):1751–60.e8.

31. Shreffler WG. Microarrayed recombinant allergens for diagnostic testing. J Allergy Clin Immunol 2011;127(4):843–9 [quiz: 850–1].

32. Nicolaou N, Poorafshar M, Murray C, et al. Allergy or tolerance in children sensitized to peanut: prevalence and differentiation using component-resolved diagnostics. J Allergy Clin Immunol 2010;125(1):191–7.e1-13.

33. Asarnoj A, Glaumann S, Elfstrom L, et al. Anaphylaxis to peanut in a patient predominantly sensitized to Ara h 6. Int Arch Allergy Immunol 2012;159(2):209–12.

34. Sicherer SH, Wood RA. Advances in diagnosing peanut allergy. J Allergy Clin Immunol Prac 2013;1(1):1–13 [quiz: 14].

35. Vereda A, van Hage M, Ahlstedt S, et al. Peanut allergy: Clinical and immunologic differences among patients from 3 different geographic regions. J Allergy Clin Immunol 2011;127(3):603–7.

36. Flinterman AE, Akkerdaas JH, den Hartog Jager CF, et al. Lipid transfer protein-linked hazelnut allergy in children from a non-Mediterranean birch-endemic area. J Allergy Clin Immunol 2008;121(2):423–8.e2.

37. Savvatianos S, Konstantinopoulos AP, Borga A, et al. Sensitization to cashew nut 2S albumin, Ana o 3, is highly predictive of cashew and pistachio allergy in Greek children. J Allergy Clin Immunol 2015;136(1):192–4.

38. Ciprandi G, Pistorio A, Silvestri M, et al. Walnut anaphylaxis: the usefulness of molecular-based allergy diagnostics. Immunol Lett 2014;161(1):138–9.

39. Le TA, Al Kindi M, Tan JA, et al. The clinical spectrum of omega-5-gliadin allergy. Intern Med J 2016;46(6):710–6.

40. Urisu A, Yamada K, Masuda S, et al. 16-kilodalton rice protein is one of the major allergens in rice grain extract and responsible for cross-allergenicity between cereal grains in the Poaceae family. Int Arch Allergy Appl Immunol 1991;96(3):244–52.

41. Battais F, Pineau F, Popineau Y, et al. Food allergy to wheat: identification of immunoglobulin E and immunoglobulin G-binding proteins with sequential extracts and purified proteins from wheat flour. Clin Exp Allergy 2003;33(7):962–70.

42. Berneder M, Bublin M, Hoffmann-Sommergruber K, et al. Allergen chip diagnosis for soy-allergic patients: Gly m 4 as a marker for severe food-allergic reactions to soy. Int Arch Allergy Immunol 2013;161(3):229–33.

43. Commins SP, Satinover SM, Hosen J, et al. Delayed anaphylaxis, angioedema, or urticaria after consumption of red meat in patients with IgE antibodies specific for galactose-alpha-1,3-galactose. J Allergy Clin Immunol 2009;123(2):426–33.

44. Hoffmann HJ, Santos AF, Mayorga C, et al. The clinical utility of basophil activation testing in diagnosis and monitoring of allergic disease. Allergy 2015;70(11):1393–405.

45. Santos AF, Brough HA. Making the most of in vitro tests to diagnose food allergy. J Allergy Clin Immunol Prac 2017;5(2):237–48.

46. Song Y, Wang J, Leung N, et al. Correlations between basophil activation, allergen-specific IgE with outcome and severity of oral food challenges. Ann Allergy Asthma Immunol 2015;114(4):319–26.
47. Hauswirth AW, Natter S, Ghannadan M, et al. Recombinant allergens promote expression of CD203c on basophils in sensitized individuals. J Allergy Clin Immunol 2002;110(1):102–9.
48. Ford LS, Bloom KA, Nowak-Wegrzyn AH, et al. Basophil reactivity, wheal size, and immunoglobulin levels distinguish degrees of cow's milk tolerance. J Allergy Clin Immunol 2013;131(1):180–6.e1-3.
49. Rubio A, Vivinus-Nebot M, Bourrier T, et al. Benefit of the basophil activation test in deciding when to reintroduce cow's milk in allergic children. Allergy 2011;66(1): 92–100.
50. Nilsson N, Nilsson C, Hedlin G, et al. Combining analyses of basophil allergen threshold sensitivity, CD-sens, and IgE antibodies to hydrolyzed wheat, omega-5 gliadin and timothy grass enhances the prediction of wheat challenge outcome. Int Arch Allergy Immunol 2013;162(1):50–7.
51. Sato S, Tachimoto H, Shukuya A, et al. Basophil activation marker CD203c is useful in the diagnosis of hen's egg and cow's milk allergies in children. Int Arch Allergy Immunol 2010;152(Suppl 1):54–61.
52. Thyagarajan A, Jones SM, Calatroni A, et al. Evidence of pathway-specific basophil anergy induced by peanut oral immunotherapy in peanut-allergic children. Clin Exp Allergy 2012;42(8):1197–205.
53. Frischmeyer-Guerrerio PA, Masilamani M, Gu W, et al. Mechanistic correlates of clinical responses to omalizumab in the setting of oral immunotherapy for milk allergy. J Allergy Clin Immunol 2017. [Epub ahead of print].
54. Vila L, Moreno A, Gamboa PM, et al. Decrease in antigen-specific CD63 basophil expression is associated with the development of tolerance to egg by SOTI in children. Pediatr Allergy Immunol 2013;24(5):463–8.
55. Jarvinen KM, Beyer K, Vila L, et al. Specificity of IgE antibodies to sequential epitopes of hen's egg ovomucoid as a marker for persistence of egg allergy. Allergy 2007;62(7):758–65.
56. Lin J, Bardina L, Shreffler WG, et al. Development of a novel peptide microarray for large-scale epitope mapping of food allergens. J Allergy Clin Immunol 2009; 124(2):315–22, 322.e1-3.
57. Jarvinen KM, Chatchatee P, Bardina L, et al. IgE and IgG binding epitopes on alpha-lactalbumin and beta-lactoglobulin in cow's milk allergy. Int Arch Allergy Immunol 2001;126(2):111–8.
58. Wang J, Lin J, Bardina L, et al. Correlation of IgE/IgG4 milk epitopes and affinity of milk-specific IgE antibodies with different phenotypes of clinical milk allergy. J Allergy Clin Immunol 2010;125(3):695–702, 702.e691-702.e696.
59. Flinterman AE, Knol EF, Lencer DA, et al. Peanut epitopes for IgE and IgG4 in peanut-sensitized children in relation to severity of peanut allergy. J Allergy Clin Immunol 2008;121(3):737–43.e10.
60. Nowak-Wegrzyn A, Assa'ad AH, Bahna SL, et al. Work Group report: oral food challenge testing. J Allergy Clin Immunol 2009;123(6 Suppl):S365–83.
61. Bird JA, Groetch M, Allen KJ, et al. Conducting an oral food challenge to peanut in an infant. J Allergy Clin Immunol Prac 2017;5(2):301–11.e1.

Food Allergy Management

Carla M. Davis, MD[a],*, John M. Kelso, MD[b]

KEYWORDS

- Management of food allergy • Epinephrine • Quality of life • Allergic reactions

KEY POINTS

- Food allergen avoidance through label reading is important to prevent accidental exposures to food.
- Prompt administration with epinephrine for anaphylaxis is associated with reduced hospitalization, morbidity, and mortality.
- Effective management of anaphylaxis in the school and community requires a comprehensive approach with adherence to a written food allergy action plan and epinephrine autoinjectors.
- Most medications and vaccines can be administered in patients with food allergy.
- Patients with food allergy at risk for poor quality of life should be given extra support through education; dietary consultation; and, in some cases, referral to a psychologist to mitigate this risk.

MANAGEMENT OF FOOD ALLERGIES

There currently is no cure for food allergies, so the management involves allergen avoidance and treatment of allergic reactions related to accidental exposure to the food. Because food is a ubiquitous part of everyday life, the allergen avoidance requirement for food allergic disease management can cause significant stress on patients and their families. However, with extensive education and physician support including practical recommendations, the stress of food allergy management is mitigated. This article discusses allergen avoidance strategies for patients with IgE- and non-IgE-mediated food allergies, medications necessary for treatment of allergic reactions, school safety laws, and factors that impact the quality of life (QoL) of patients with food allergy. Potential nutritional deficiencies and the risk of reactions to vaccines and other medications associated with specific food allergies are discussed.

FOOD ALLERGEN AVOIDANCE

Current management of food allergies relies on the careful elimination of the offending food from the diet and, in IgE-mediated disease, the prompt institution of therapeutic

[a] Section of Immunology, Allergy and Rheumatology, Baylor College of Medicine, Texas Children's Hospital, 1102 Bates Avenue, MC 330.01, Houston, TX 77030, USA; [b] Division of Allergy, Asthma and Immunology, Scripps Clinic, 3811 Valley Centre Drive, San Diego, CA 92130, USA
* Corresponding author.
E-mail addresses: carlad@bcm.edu; cmdavis@texaschildrens.org

Immunol Allergy Clin N Am 38 (2018) 53–64
https://doi.org/10.1016/j.iac.2017.09.005
0889-8561/18/© 2017 Elsevier Inc. All rights reserved.

immunology.theclinics.com

measures to treat severe reactions in cases of accidental exposure. Follow-up with a physician is required after a severe food allergic reaction for observation for 4 to 6 hours to monitor for biphasic reactions, such as anaphylaxis, which can occur in 0.6% to 15% of cases.[1,2] These treatment measures are not required in non-IgE-mediated reactions because these delayed chronic conditions rarely evolve into acute life-threatening reactions (**Table 1**). However, food elimination from the diet is still important in non-IgE-mediated disease to prevent delayed symptoms. Because IgE-mediated disease is life threatening, food allergen exposure through cross-contact or cross-contamination is more important in this disease compared with non-IgE-mediated disease.

Elimination of offending foods from the diet sounds like a trivial exercise, but because of often surprising uses of various food products in industrial food preparation processes and problems of cross-contamination in food-processing facilities, this is challenging. Instruction about the fastidious avoidance of specific allergens by reading of labels (note that the components of commercial food products often change without notice) requires education of the parents by a dietitian or other provider with specific expertise in appropriate counseling of families, such as an allergist. Instructions should be given in oral and written form for each patient.

The Food Allergen Labeling and Consumer Protection Act (FALCPA) was passed to assist consumers with food allergy in the avoidance of products with specific food allergens.[3] It is an amendment to the Federal Food, Drug, and Cosmetic Act and requires that the label of a food that contains an ingredient that is or contains protein from a "major food allergen" declare the presence of the allergen in the manner described by the law. The allergens included in the act are milk, egg, soy, wheat, tree nut, peanut, shrimp, fish, and soybeans. However, there are limitations to the Act, discussed later.[4]

All foods that contain even trace amounts of these allergens should be avoided by individuals with food allergy.[5] Cross-contact or cross-contamination of safe foods with a patient's known allergen should be avoided. More than 160 foods have been identified to cause food allergies in sensitive individuals. There are other common allergens that are not included in the FALCPA list.[4] Patients allergic to sesame should be told that sesame and other seeds are not included on the allergen labeling. The best advice for patients with food allergy is to avoid eating the food if the ingredients are unknown. In children, elimination diets carry a risk of inducing malnutrition with poor growth because of the elimination of essential nutrients. In cases of multiple food allergies, monitoring by an experienced pediatric dietitian to ensure adequate nutrient intake is useful.

There are patient advocacy organizations that provide written and online information about label reading that is useful for patients and families (eg, Food Allergy Research and Education, www.foodallergy.org). The written material should include

Table 1	
Food allergic disorders	
Acute Onset (IgE Mediated)	**Delayed Onset (IgE and/or Cellular Mediated)**
Urticaria/angioedema	Atopic dermatitis
Anaphylaxis	Eosinophilic esophagitis and other
Oral allergy syndrome	eosinophilic gastroenteropathies
Food-associated, exercise-induced	Food protein–induced enterocolitis syndrome
anaphylaxis	Allergic proctocolitis
Alpha gal mammalian meat allergy	Contact dermatitis

terms that are used to designate specific food allergen–containing ingredients. Many of these words may not be recognizable to patients or their families. For example, caseinates, ghee, or nisin may be label ingredient terms for milk-containing products or einkorn, durum, or kamut may be label ingredient terms for wheat-containing products. These milk and wheat derivatives are still covered by FALCPA,[3] so "milk" or "wheat" appear on the label. Patients with food allergy should be educated about obscure words for a pertinent allergen they may encounter during label reading in case they are traveling out of the country or eating packaged foods with allergens not covered under FALCPA.

CLINICAL SYMPTOMS OF REACTIONS TO FOOD ALLERGENS

Food allergies are grouped in two general categories: IgE-mediated and non-IgE-mediated (see **Table 1**). IgE-mediated reactions are typically of rapid onset with clinical symptoms usually developing within minutes to a few hours of ingestion of the offending food. These reactions exhibit a characteristic pattern of a type I hypersensitivity reaction, mediated by mast cell and basophil degranulation. Skin manifestations (ie, flushing, urticaria, and/or angioedema) occur in more than two-thirds of affected children, but some may present with respiratory or gastrointestinal manifestations exclusively (**Table 2**).[6,7] Progression to full-blown anaphylaxis with cardiovascular collapse may occur.

An IgE-triggered reaction in the oral mucosa underlies oral allergy syndrome, in which subjects complain of pruritus of the mouth and/or throat when they eat raw vegetables and fruits. This syndrome develops exclusively in the older child or teenager with prior pollen sensitization and is caused by heat-labile cross-reactive antigens present in plant and food antigens.[5,6] Usually, these foods are well tolerated when cooked.

Delayed reactions to mammalian meat 3 to 6 hours after ingestion are caused by an IgE-mediated reaction to the carbohydrate antigen galactose-alpha-1,3-galactose (also known as "alpha gal"), a sugar moiety lining the surface of nonprimate mammalian tissue. Allergic reactions to beef, lamb, and pork are caused by IgE to alpha gal. The production of the alpha gal IgE is triggered by tick bites so many patients with delayed reactions to mammalian meat have a prior history of tick bites.[1]

Table 2
Clinical manifestations of food hypersensitivity

Cutaneous	Respiratory	Gastrointestinal	Cardiovascular	Neurologic/Other
Urticaria	Rhinorrhea	Abdominal pain	Loss of consciousness	Lethargy
Flushing	Swelling of lips, tongue, and/or throat	Dysphagia	Hypotension	Headache
Angioedema	Cough	Emesis	Shock	Anxiety
Atopic dermatitis	Wheeze or stridor	Diarrhea	Tachycardia or bradycardia	Confusion
Contact dermatitis	Shortness of breath	Hematochezia		Lightheadedness
Pruritus	Pain with swallowing	Malabsorption		Loss of bladder control
	Hoarseness	Failure to thrive		Pelvic pain

In non-IgE-mediated food hypersensitivity reactions, T cell–mediated mechanisms provide the predominant pathogenic stimulus that drives the clinical manifestations. In some, there may be findings of concomitant sensitization (ie, detection of food-specific IgE), but symptoms of a type I hypersensitivity reaction as such are usually absent. T cell–mediated delayed hypersensitivity (T helper cell 2 responses) has been suggested as a cause of delayed onset of inflammation in patients with atopic dermatitis and eosinophilic esophagitis.[6]

Food allergy contributes to the development of atopic dermatitis in the pediatric age group. Allergies exacerbate atopic dermatitis in about one-third of cases. Infants and young children may exhibit worsening symptoms when exposed to particular foods, either directly or through breast milk. Atopic dermatitis onset is most common at 3 to 6 months of age and food-specific IgE is highest in infants who develop eczema within the first 3 months of age. Atopic dermatitis flares can occur within hours or days of exposure to foods in susceptible patients. The rash usually improves following an elimination of known food allergens. However, there is little evidence that use of exclusion diet in unselected individuals with atopic eczema is useful.[6]

Urticaria and angioedema are typical of mild food allergic reactions. Urticaria and angioedema are localized swelling of the skin or mucous membranes. Urticaria, commonly called hives, involves extravasation of fluid in the superficial dermis. It is characterized by well-circumscribed, pruritic, raised erythematous skin wheals, often with central pallor and blanching with applied pressure. Angioedema results from similar vasopermeability in the deeper layers of the dermis and subcutaneous tissue. Angioedema may appear associated with urticaria, but occasionally presents as an isolated symptom. Angioedema typically involves the periorbital tissues, lips, tongue, posterior oropharynx, larynx, hands, feet, or genitals. Less commonly, angioedema may involve the gastrointestinal tract, resulting in abdominal pain, nausea, vomiting, and diarrhea. Edematous swelling of angioedema may take 24 to 72 hours, or in some instances longer, to fully resolve.[8]

During reactions, if the reaction only involves hives or angioedema of the skin, and does not involve the posterior oropharynx or larynx, causing difficulty breathing, this reaction is considered mild. Other symptoms consistent with mild reactions are gastrointestinal symptoms, such as nausea and mild abdominal pain. These are treated with an H_1 antihistamine, such as diphenhydramine, or with an H_2 antihistamine if indicated. If a mild food allergic reaction progresses, treatment other than antihistamine is required. Epinephrine should be given if the patient develops anaphylactic symptoms. Anaphylaxis is the most severe food allergic reaction and is diagnosed when there are two body systems involved in a reaction or if there is respiratory and/or cardiovascular compromise (**Box 1**). The criteria to diagnose this has been validated and should be used as a guide for treatment with epinephrine.[9]

MANAGEMENT OF FOOD ALLERGIC REACTIONS

All patients with a history of a systemic allergic reaction to food should be prescribed self-injectable epinephrine with a formulation appropriate for the patient's weight and instructed on its use. A written plan outlining the symptoms requiring epinephrine use can facilitate appropriate treatment. This drug should be used promptly in the case of an impending anaphylactic reaction. Patients should carry two doses at all times because biphasic reactions can occur and one epinephrine dose may not halt symptom progression. A second dose should be given if the reaction is progressive. Milder reactions are managed with oral H_1 and H_2 antihistamines. β_2-Agonists and glucocorticoids are used as second-line agents.[6,7]

Box 1
Criteria for anaphylaxis diagnosis

Anaphylaxis is highly likely when any one of the following three criteria is fulfilled:

Acute onset of an illness (minutes to several hours), with involvement of the skin, mucosal tissue, or both (eg, generalized urticaria, itching or flushing, swollen lips/tongue/uvula), and at least one of the following: (1) respiratory compromise (eg, dyspnea, wheeze/bronchospasm, stridor, hypoxemia) or (2) reduced blood pressure or associated symptoms of end-organ dysfunction (eg, hypotonia [collapse], syncope, incontinence).

Two or more of the following that occur suddenly after exposure to a likely allergen for that patient (minutes to several hours): (1) involvement of the skin/mucosal tissue (eg, generalized urticaria, itch/flush, swollen lips/tongue/uvula), (2) respiratory compromise (eg, dyspnea, wheeze/bronchospasm, stridor, hypoxemia), (3) reduced blood pressure or associated symptoms (eg, hypotonia [collapse], syncope, incontinence), or (4) persistent gastrointestinal symptoms (eg, crampy abdominal pain, vomiting).

Reduced blood pressure after exposure to a known allergen for that patient (minutes to several hours): (1) for infants and children, low systolic blood pressure (age-specific) or greater than 30% decrease in systolic blood pressure, and (2) for teenagers and adults, systolic blood pressure of less than 90 mm Hg or greater than 30% decrease from that person's baseline.

Adapted from Sampson HA, Muñoz-Furlong A, Campbell RL, et al. Second symposium on the definition and management of anaphylaxis: summary report—Second National Institute of Allergy and Infectious Disease/Food Allergy and Anaphylaxis Network symposium. J Allergy Clin Immunol 2006;117(2):393; with permission.

Epinephrine

The first-line therapy for severe food allergic reactions is epinephrine. In IgE-mediated food allergies, exposure to a trace amount of food allergen may trigger a severe allergic reaction or anaphylaxis. These reactions can be life threatening and, in rare cases, result in death. The approach to treating anaphylaxis should focus first on maintaining the airway, breathing, and circulation. Mortality from anaphylaxis results from asphyxiation caused by upper airway angioedema, respiratory failure from severe bronchial obstruction, or cardiovascular collapse. Epinephrine is most effective when administered within 30 minutes of symptom onset.[10] Anaphylaxis mortality is strongly correlated with delays in epinephrine therapy.

Hypotension requires aggressive large-volume fluid resuscitation and, if persistent, vasopressor therapy. Supplemental oxygen is recommended, and in the presence of respiratory compromise or bronchospasm, inhaled bronchodilators, such as albuterol, should be administered. Intubation and mechanical ventilation may be necessary. Anaphylactic reactions that occur in patients taking β-adrenergic antagonists may be particularly refractory to epinephrine. In this setting, glucagon or atropine administration should be considered. Whenever possible, patients should be observed for 4 to 6 hours after an anaphylactic reaction because of the possibility of recurrent symptoms from the late-phase response occurring several hours after the initial event.

All patients should be discharged with injectable epinephrine for home use after an anaphylactic event, ensuring that they receive appropriate instruction in the use of an auto injector of epinephrine.[11] Subsequent to treatment of the acute episode, identification of the triggering antigen or exposure should be pursued through diagnostic allergy skin testing or serum IgE testing whenever possible. Patients should strongly consider wearing medical alert identification detailing their specific allergies if known.

In the community, epinephrine should be given promptly with intramuscular epinephrine injection in the mid-outer thigh. An autoinjector is the best device to administer this medication. This can reduce hospitalizations, morbidity, and mortality. Autoinjectable epinephrine should be given by prescription to patients with food allergy at risk for life-threatening anaphylaxis to carry with them when they reach an age of responsibility. The injectors should be kept at room temperature and each patient should practice using the trainer device to become comfortable with its use.[12]

Antihistamines

Histamine is a primary amine produced by mast cells and basophils that orchestrates many aspects of the allergic response by binding to specific receptors present on the surface of its target cells. So far, four types of histamine receptors belonging to the G protein–coupled receptor family have been identified: H_1, H_2, H_3, and H_4. Signals transduced via the H_1 (and to a lesser extent H_2) receptor mediate many of the acute symptoms and signs of allergic disease in the skin, airway, and gastrointestinal tract, whereas H_1 and H_4 seem to promote the accumulation of inflammatory cells at sites of allergic inflammation.[13]

Histamine receptor antagonists are prescribed for the treatment of allergic reactions. Oral H_1 antihistamine reduces responses to allergen in the conjunctiva, nose, and skin, and administering the drug during the course of an allergic response curbs the symptoms triggered by mild acute allergic inflammation. Onset of action occurs within minutes to 1 to 3 hours. Newer H_1 antihistamines have a prolonged half-life and need to be administered only once or twice daily for continued allergic symptoms. Shorter acting antihistamines have to be administered every 4 to 6 hours to maintain efficacy for continued symptoms. Symptom relief may be insufficient when other mediators (eg, leukotrienes, neuropeptides) are involved. This is often the case in the pruritus of atopic dermatitis, which, by and large, is resistant to antihistamines.[13] Additionally, anaphylaxis should not be treated with antihistamines instead of epinephrine because multiple mediators are involved. Epinephrine is the first-line treatment of anaphylaxis.[14]

Adjuvant Therapies

Corticosteroids are pleiotropic anti-inflammatory drugs with proven efficacy in the management of various aspects of allergic inflammation. The development of highly effective topical preparations (intranasal, inhaled, or dermatologic creams) with minimal systemic effects has revolutionized the therapy for common disorders, such as allergic rhinitis, allergic asthma, and atopic dermatitis. For food allergic reactions, steroids are frequently used as an adjuvant therapy to attenuate the potential late-phase inflammatory response after anaphylaxis. However, steroids have not been proven to prevent biphasic responses after a primary anaphylactic reaction. Inhaled β_2-agonist medications are also given as adjuvant treatment of patients with food allergy with wheezing and cough during an anaphylactic reaction to help relieve pulmonary bronchoconstriction. The use of albuterol should not delay the use of epinephrine as the primary treatment of food-induced anaphylaxis.[13,14]

School Management of Food Allergies

Students with food allergies spend most of their day in a school setting. In addition, because 1 to 2 students out of 30 children have food allergies,[5] the school setting should be focused on safety for the children with life-threatening allergies. The student with an undiagnosed food allergy may experience his or her first food allergy reaction at school. Studies regarding epinephrine administration show that almost one in four administrations of epinephrine involved a student whose allergy was unknown by the school at the time of his or her reaction.[15]

It is helpful for a school to adopt a state or national guideline to managing life-threatening food allergies in their students. Effective management of anaphylaxis in the school and community requires a comprehensive approach involving children, families, preschools, schools, camps, universities, and sports organizations. A practical method of involving all stakeholders in a school for the safety of a child with food allergy is to have a team meeting of all persons involved in that child's care during the day to talk about the food avoidance plan, recognition of allergic reactions, and prompt treatment of accidental exposure. This should occur before the child is enrolled or immediately after an allergic reaction. An important component of effective management of food allergies in schools includes a written, personalized anaphylaxis emergency action plan with the trigger food allergen clearly noted on the plan. School administration and nursing coordination are helpful to facilitate communication among the child's providers during the day.[1,12,15]

Current federal laws are helpful in managing food allergies in schools. When a physician assesses that a child's food allergy may result in anaphylaxis, the child's condition meets the definition of "disability" and is covered under federal laws, such as the Americans with Disabilities Act (ADA), Section 504 of the Rehabilitation Act of 1973, and possibly the Individuals with Disabilities Education Act (IDEA) if the allergy management affects the student's ability to make educational progress.[15]

The IDEA assists States and school districts in making a "free appropriate public education" available to eligible students. Under IDEA, a "free appropriate public education" means special education and related services provided under public supervision and direction, in conformity with an individualized education program, at no cost to parents. A student who has a food allergy and who is making effective educational progress in the regular education program has the right to have the school make reasonable accommodations for his or her disability, under section 504 and the ADA.[15]

Title II of the ADA, enacted in 1990, prohibits discrimination against qualified individuals with life-threatening food allergies in state and local government programs and services, including public schools. Title III of the ADA extends requirements for public accommodations to privately owned facilities. Thus, all private schools participating in the federally funded child nutrition programs must make accommodations to enable children with life-threatening food allergies to receive school meals.[15]

Under the USDA Federal Regulation "Exceptions for medical or special dietary needs" law (7 CFR 210.10 [1]), schools must make substitutions in lunches and afterschool snacks for students who are considered to have a disability under 7 CFR part 15b and whose disability restricts their diet. Schools may also make substitutions for students who do not have a disability but who cannot consume the regular lunch or afterschool snack because of medical or other special dietary needs. Substitutions must be made on a case by case basis only when supported by a statement of the need for substitutions that includes recommended alternate foods, unless otherwise exempted. Such statements must, in the case of a student with a disability, be signed by a physician or, in the case of a student who is not disabled, by a recognized medical authority.[15]

FOOD ALLERGENS IN MEDICATIONS AND VACCINES

Certain excipients used in medications and vaccines are derived from food.[16] Providers and patients and parents of children with food allergy may wonder whether or not it is safe to take medications or receive immunizations containing these food-derived excipients. Although there are exceptions, in most cases, the use of these products is safe because the excipients contain little if any food protein.[16] A few of the more common food allergies where questions have arisen about specific medications are reviewed next.

Milk

Casamino acids

The growth media for diphtheria, tetanus, and pertussis–containing vaccines (DTaP and Tdap) contain amino acids derived from the milk protein casein. There are rare reports of children exquisitely allergic to milk who have had anaphylactic reactions to these vaccines attributed to contaminating milk proteins.[17] Given the uneventful near universal vaccination of millions of children with milk allergy, such reactions are rare. Patients with milk allergy need not avoid these vaccines.[18] However, in the rare patient with milk allergy who has an apparent allergic reaction to such a vaccine, it is appropriate to perform skin testing with the suspect vaccine and another lot and, if positive, consider evaluation for contaminating milk proteins.

Lactose

Lactose is milk sugar purified from cow's milk. Pharmaceutical-grade lactose is usually free of contaminating milk proteins and most patients with milk allergy have negative skin tests and oral challenges to lactose.[19] Rarely, lactose is contaminated with milk proteins and causes reactions in patients allergic to milk. Most dry powder inhalers (DPIs) contain lactose to improve drug delivery and to impart taste to indicate dose delivery. There are isolated reports of patients who had asthma symptoms immediately after use of a DPI, and milk proteins were detected in the suspect lot of medication but not in different lots.[16] This is clearly a rare phenomenon given the large number of children with milk allergy who use lactose-containing DPIs uneventfully. Patients with milk allergy need not avoid lactose-containing DPIs. However, in the rare patient with milk allergy who reported such an exacerbation with a DPI, it is appropriate to perform skin testing with the suspect DPI and another lot and, if positive, consider evaluation for contaminating milk proteins.

Egg

Ovalbumin

Although most injectable inactivated influenza vaccines (IIV) and the intranasally administered live attenuated influenza vaccine (LAIV) are grown in eggs and contain measurable quantities of egg protein (ovalbumin), research studies involving thousands of recipients allergic to egg including hundreds with anaphylactic sensitivity to the ingestion of egg have demonstrated no increase in the rate of allergy-like events compared with recipients not allergic to egg,[20] likely due to there being insufficient egg protein in these vaccines to elicit an allergic response even in the most exquisitely allergic subjects. As a result, the American Academy of Pediatrics' Committee on Infectious Diseases has stated that all children with egg allergy can receive influenza vaccine with no additional precautions from those of routine vaccinations; that IIV administered in a single, age-appropriate dose is well tolerated by recipients with a history of egg allergy of any severity; that egg allergy does not impart an increased risk of anaphylactic reaction to vaccination with IIV; and that LAIV is well tolerated in children with a history of anaphylaxis after exposure to egg, similar to IIV.[21] Thus, vaccine providers need not inquire about the egg allergy status of influenza vaccine recipients.

Egg lecithin

Lecithin is a fatty substance derived most often for use as a pharmaceutical excipient from egg and soy and does contain residual amounts of protein.[22] Concern about its use has been raised most often in regard to propofol, an intravenous sedative-hypnotic agent used in anesthesia that is formulated in a fat emulsion containing soybean oil and egg lecithin.[23] There are reports of patients with apparent anaphylactic reactions to propofol. However, most have occurred in patients without egg allergy, and most patients with egg allergy receive propofol uneventfully.[24] Thus, although propofol can cause anaphylactic reactions, the mechanism is unclear and seems unrelated to egg or soy allergy.[16] Patients allergic to egg need not avoid propofol or other medications containing egg lecithin.

Fish and Shellfish

Protamine is a small protein involved in sperm biology. For pharmaceutical use, it is isolated from salmon testes and used to reverse heparin and complexed to insulin to delay absorption.[25] Urticarial and anaphylactic reactions to protamine have been reported. A few of these reports have been in patients with fish allergy, suggesting cross-reactions with other fish proteins.[16] However, enzyme-linked immunosorbent assay inhibition with sera from patients with salmon allergy showed no inhibition with protamine and most patients with fish allergy tolerate protamine uneventfully.[26,27] Thus, although protamine can cause anaphylactic reactions, the mechanism is unclear and seems unrelated to fish allergy.[16] Thus, patients with fish allergy do not need to avoid protamine.

Glucosamine is an amino sugar derived from the shells of shellfish and is used as a food supplement purportedly to relieve joint pain. Although there are rare reports of possibly allergic reactions to glucosamine, they have not been in subjects allergic to shellfish and patients with documented shellfish allergy tolerate glucosamine uneventfully.[16] Thus, patients with shellfish allergy do not need to avoid glucosamine.

Soy

Soy lecithin is also used as a pharmaceutical excipient. There are few reports of asthma exacerbations or other potentially allergic reactions after the use of ipratropium metered-dose inhalers containing soy lecithin in patients allergic to soy; however, none describe any testing to support the notion that the reactions were caused by contaminating soy protein.[16] Despite this lack of evidence or any evidence of cross-reactivity, the package inserts for these products extended this precaution to "related food products such as soybean or peanut," which seems wholly unwarranted. Nonetheless, current formulations of these products do not contain soy lecithin. Thus, there are no inhalers that need to be avoided by patients with soy or other food allergy.

Gelatin

Gelatin is produced by partial hydrolysis of collagen from cows or pigs and contains potentially allergenic protein fragments. Bovine and porcine gelatins are extensively cross-reactive, but do not cross-react with plant and fish gelatins.[16] Gelatin is added to many (especially live attenuated viral) vaccines as a stabilizer and is responsible for many anaphylactic reactions to these vaccines.[28] Parenterally administered vaccines available in the United States that contain gelatin include LAIV, mumps-measles-rubella, Purified chick embryo cell (PCEC) rabies vaccine, varicella, yellow fever, and zoster.

Although reports of allergic reactions to medications in gelatin-containing capsules are rare, there are reports of absorption from mucosal surfaces causing anaphylaxis including from suppositories[29] and hemostatic sponges.[30,31] In addition, outside the

United States, gelatin solutions are used as intravenous volume expanders and there are numerous reports of anaphylactic reactions to these.[16]

Thus, there are many well-documented cases of IgE-mediated anaphylactic reactions to gelatin contained in medications, vaccines, and other medical products. Patients with gelatin allergy should generally avoid such products. A history of allergy to the ingestion of gelatin should be sought before the administration of such products. However, a negative history may not exclude an allergic reaction to gelatin administered by injection or applied to mucosal surfaces where it is absorbed without digestion. Thus, if the patient suffers an apparent allergic reaction after receipt of a gelatin-containing medication or vaccine, they should be evaluated for gelatin allergy.[16]

In summary, it is clear that, with the exception of gelatin, most patients with food allergy can tolerate medications containing excipients derived from the foods to which they are allergic without reaction because such excipients contain no or not enough (micrograms or less) contaminating protein to provoke a reaction. These patients should be advised that they need not avoid such products. In the rare circumstance where a patient with food allergy reacts to a medical product containing a food-derived excipient, it should still not be assumed that the product caused the reaction without demonstrating that the suspect product contains contaminating protein. The reason that gelatin-containing products are more likely to cause reactions in subjects allergic to gelatin is likely because of the much larger quantity (milligrams or more) of protein in these products, and these patients should be advised to avoid such products, or, in the case of vaccines, consider having them administered in graded doses under observation.[28]

QUALITY OF LIFE PREDICTORS

Food allergy impacts the QoL of patients, their families, and social contacts. There are considerable detrimental effects of the burden of living with food allergies. These include an increased financial burden from food purchases, increased food preparation time, anxiety and fear of accidental exposure and allergic reactions, burden of constant vigilance to avoid allergens, and social isolation from restricted activities. Certain groups are more likely to be affected than others. Mothers have more burden of responsibility to keep a child with food allergy safe than fathers, causing lower QoL. Caregivers with more than one child and caregivers of a child allergic to more than one food were more at risk of lower QoL. Females with food allergy and people with a higher number of previous reactions or atopic diseases have lower QoL than their counterparts.[32]

Physicians should be aware of the qualities of patients with food allergy who are at risk of lower QoL. Although not validated, education of the rare risk of death from anaphylaxis when prompt treatment is administered, community education efforts through school personnel training, and development of communication skills with role playing for small children are some strategies that may be beneficial for improving QoL in these patients. Occasionally, psychology referral is necessary to provide additional support.[32]

FUTURE ALLERGEN-SPECIFIC IMMUNOTHERAPY

Allergen-specific subcutaneous immunotherapy has been practiced since the late 1950s and has proven to be clearly effective therapy for allergic airway diseases but was associated with severe life-threatening reactions with administration of food allergens by this route. The use of less invasive methods, such as oral, sublingual, and epicutaneous immunotherapy for desensitization to food allergens, is currently an area of intense investigation. The latter three routes of immunotherapy cause some degree of desensitization, with oral being the most effective. However, the risk of systemic reactions and gastrointestinal symptoms are highest with oral immunotherapy. So, although promising, the risk of reactions during treatment compared with the therapeutic benefit for food oral immunotherapy has yet to be established as favorable in infants and children. In the future, lessons learned from these studies are likely to result in improved treatment of food allergies.[33]

Effective management of food allergies includes a multifaceted approach. This includes patient education of the need for strict food allergen avoidance to prevent accidental exposures, prompt administration of epinephrine for anaphylaxis, and a comprehensive school-based plan with written food allergy action plans and access to epinephrine autoinjectors. Most medications and vaccines can be administered in patients with food allergy. Patients with food allergy at risk for poor QoL should be given extra support through education; dietary consultation; and, in appropriate cases, referral to a psychologist.

REFERENCES

1. Sicherer SH, Sampson HA. Food allergy: epidemiology, pathogenesis, diagnosis, and treatment. J Allergy Clin Immunol 2014;133:291–307.

2. Katz Y, Nowak-Węgrzyn A, Spergel JM. Prevalence of biphasic response in anaphylaxis due to purposeful administration of allergenic food. Ann Allergy Asthma Immunol 2015;115(6):526–7.

3. Thompson T, Kane RR, Hager MH. Food allergen labeling and consumer protection act of 2004 in effect. J Am Diet Assoc 2006;106(11):1742–4.

4. Gendel SM, Zhu J. Analysis of U.S. Food and Drug Administration food allergen recalls after implementation of the food allergen labeling and consumer protection act. J Food Prot 2013;76(11):1933–8.

5. Boyce JA, Assa'ad A, Burks AW, et al. Guidelines for the diagnosis and management of food allergy in the United States: report of the NIAID-sponsored expert panel. J Allergy Clin Immunol 2010;126:S1–58.

6. Sampson HA, Aceves S, Bock SA, et al. Food allergy: a practice parameter update-2014. J Allergy Clin Immunol 2014;134:1016–25.e43.

7. Nowak-Wegrzyn A, Assa'ad AH, Bahna SL, et al. Work group report: oral food challenge testing. J Allergy Clin Immunol 2009;123(6 Suppl):S365.

8. Baxi S, Dinakar C. Urticaria and angioedema. Immunol Allergy Clin North Am 2005;25:353–67, 15878460.

9. Sampson HA, Muñoz-Furlong A, Campbell RL, et al. Second symposium on the definition and management of anaphylaxis: summary report—Second National Institute of Allergy and Infectious Disease/Food Allergy and Anaphylaxis Network Symposium. J Allergy Clin Immunol 2006;117(2):391–7.

10. Kemp SF, Lockey RF, Simons FE, et al. Epinephrine: the drug of choice for anaphylaxis. A statement of the World Allergy Organization. Allergy 2008;63:1061–70.

11. Mehr S, Robinson M, Tang M. Doctor—how do I use my EpiPen? Pediatr Allergy Immunol 2007;18:448–52.

12. Sicherer SH, Simons FER, Section on allergy and immunology. Epinephrine for first-aid management of anaphylaxis. Pediatrics 2017;139(3) [pii:e20164006].

13. Garcia-Lloret M. Clinical aspects of allergic diseases. In: Rudolph C, Rudolph A, Lister G, et al, editors. Rudolph's pediatrics. 22nd edition. Appleton & Lange; 2011.

14. Riedl M. Anaphylaxis, urticaria, and angioedema. In: Rudolph C, Rudolph A, Lister G, et al, editors. Rudolph's pediatrics. 22nd edition. Appleton & Lange; 2011.

15. Young MC, Muñoz-Furlong A, Sicherer SH. Management of food allergies in schools: a perspective for allergists. J Allergy Clin Immunol 2009;124(2):175–82.

16. Kelso JM. Potential food allergens in medications. J Allergy Clin Immunol 2014; 133:1509–18.

17. Kattan JD, Konstantinou GN, Cox AL, et al. Anaphylaxis to diphtheria, tetanus, and pertussis vaccines among children with cow's milk allergy. J Allergy Clin Immunol 2011;128(1):215–8.

18. Slater JE, Rabin RL, Martin D. Comments on cow's milk allergy and diphtheria, tetanus, and pertussis vaccines. J Allergy Clin Immunol 2011;128:434.

19. Fiocchi A, Restani P, Leo G, et al. Clinical tolerance to lactose in children with cow's milk allergy. Pediatrics 2003;112:359–62.

20. Kelso JM. Administering influenza vaccine to egg-allergic persons. Expert Rev Vaccin 2014;13:1049–57.

21. Committee on Infectious Diseases. Recommendations for prevention and control of influenza in children, 2016-2017. Pediatrics 2016;138(4) [pii:e20162527].

22. Martin-Hernandez C, Benet S, Marvin-Guy LF. Characterization and quantification of proteins in lecithins. J Agric Food Chem 2005;53:8607–13.

23. AstraZeneca Pharmaceuticals L. DIPRIVAN - propofol injection, emulsion [package insert]. Wilmington (DE): AstraZeneca Pharmaceuticals; 2005.

24. Murphy A, Campbell DE, Baines D, et al. Allergic reactions to propofol in egg-allergic children. Anesth Analg 2011;113:140–4.

25. Joint Task Force on Practice Parameters, American Academy of Allergy, Asthma and Immunology, American College of Allergy, Asthma and Immunology, Joint Council of Allergy, Asthma and Immunology. Drug allergy: an updated practice parameter. Ann Allergy Asthma Immunol 2010;105:259–73.

26. Greenberger PA, Patterson R, Tobin MC, et al. Lack of cross-reactivity between IgE to salmon and protamine sulfate. Am J Med Sci 1989;298:104–8.

27. Levy JH, Schwieger IM, Zaidan JR, et al. Evaluation of patients at risk for protamine reactions. J Thorac Cardiovasc Surg 1989;98:200–4.

28. Dreskin SC, Halsey NA, Kelso JM, et al. International Consensus (ICON): allergic reactions to vaccines. World Allergy Organ J 2016;9:1–21.

29. Sakaguchi M, Inouye S. Anaphylaxis to gelatin-containing rectal suppositories. J Allergy Clin Immunol 2001;108:1033–4.

30. Khoriaty E, McClain CD, Permaul P, et al. Intraoperative anaphylaxis induced by the gelatin component of thrombin-soaked gelfoam in a pediatric patient. Ann Allergy Asthma Immunol 2012;108:209–10.

31. Spencer HT, Hsu JT, McDonald DR, et al. Intraoperative anaphylaxis to gelatin in topical hemostatic agents during anterior spinal fusion: a case report. Spine J 2012;12:e1–6.

32. Cummings AJ, Knibb RC, King RM, et al. The psychosocial impact of food allergy and food hypersensitivity in children, adolescents and their families: a review. Allergy 2010;65(8):933–45.

33. Wood RA. Food allergen immunotherapy: current status and prospects for the future. J Allergy Clin Immunol 2016;137:973–82.

The Role of Baked Egg and Milk in the Diets of Allergic Children

Melissa L. Robinson, DO[a,b,*], Bruce J. Lanser, MD[b,c]

KEYWORDS

- Food allergy • Egg allergy • Milk allergy • Baked egg • Baked milk • Immunotherapy
- Eosinophilic esophagitis

KEY POINTS

- Most children with an immunoglobulin E–mediated food allergy to egg or cow's milk can tolerate these foods in baked form.
- Eating baked goods containing egg or cow's milk may hasten the development of tolerance to these foods in an unheated form.
- Given the poor performance of standard allergy sensitization tests for baked egg and baked milk tolerance, most patients with egg or milk allergy should be considered for an oral food challenge to baked goods.
- Diets containing egg and milk in baked goods are well-tolerated after passing a challenge and can improve the quality of life for families with food allergy.

INTRODUCTION

Hen's egg and cow's milk (CM) allergy are the most prevalent immunoglobulin E (IgE)–mediated food allergies in young children, affecting up to 1.8% of children younger than 5 years.[1] The current standard-of-care recommendations for IgE-mediated food allergy include strict dietary avoidance of the food in all forms, education, and recognition of reactions.[2] Patients must also carry rescue medication at all times and should always have an epinephrine autoinjector available when eating any foods. Various forms of immunotherapy for egg and CM remain under investigation, with some promising preliminary results; but this is not yet considered part of routine clinical practice, as more research is required.[3]

Disclosure Statement: Both authors have no relevant financial relationships to disclose.
[a] Department of Pediatrics, National Jewish Health, 1400 Jackson Street, K830, Denver, CO 80206, USA; [b] Department of Pediatrics, University of Colorado School of Medicine, Aurora, CO, USA; [c] Department of Pediatrics, Division of Allergy and Clinical Immunology, National Jewish Health, 1400 Jackson Street, J322, Denver, CO 80206, USA
* Corresponding author. 1400 Jackson Street, K830, Denver, CO 80206.
E-mail address: Robinsonm2@njhealth.org

Immunol Allergy Clin N Am 38 (2018) 65–76
https://doi.org/10.1016/j.iac.2017.09.007
0889-8561/18/© 2017 Elsevier Inc. All rights reserved.

immunology.theclinics.com

Egg and CM are found in an abundance of foods across many cultures, particularly in baked and/or processed products. This dietary restriction can be difficult with increased psychosocial burden and risks of inadequate nutrient intake in egg- and CM-allergic children.[4] Both egg and CM allergy have a good prognosis, with most children outgrowing their allergy.[5,6] However, it seems that tolerance is taking longer to develop than previously observed, with egg and CM allergies persisting longer into adolescence and adulthood.[7,8] Several studies have demonstrated that the incorporation of egg and CM in baked form into the diets of allergic children offers several benefits: it may accelerate the development of tolerance to unheated egg and CM, enhance the quality of life for the child and family via liberalization of the diet, and improve nutritional status.[4] Diets containing egg and CM in baked goods may represent a safe and well-tolerated alternative form of oral immunotherapy (OIT) with similar immunologic changes that are observed in OIT clinical trials.

ALTERING THE ALLERGENICITY OF MILK AND EGG

In both egg and CM allergy, food processing alters the allergenicity of various proteins within the food. Heating denatures the structure of heat-labile food proteins. With the destruction of heat-labile proteins, the IgE binding sites may be altered and affect the ability for food-specific IgE antibodies to bind. This decreased binding and allergenicity of baked egg and baked CM may permit individuals to eat and tolerate baked egg and baked CM without adverse reactions, despite continued sensitivity to unheated egg and CM.

In egg white (EW), the proteins ovalbumin (Gal d I) and ovomucoid (OVM, Gal d III) are the predominant allergens but have different levels of heat susceptibility.[9] Ovalbumin is the most abundant protein fraction in egg and is heat sensitive with resultant decreased allergenicity.[10,11] In contrast, OVM is thought to be the major allergen and is heat resistant; however, when OVM is complexed with gluten in wheat and sufficiently baked, it is largely unable to be bound by egg specific IgE (sIgE).[12] In a clinical study, Urisu and colleagues[12] demonstrated decreased allergenicity during oral food challenges (OFCs) with heated and OVM-depleted egg compared with heated egg in individuals with high sIgE values to EW.[11]

Similar to egg protein, CM proteins are denatured with high heat. The predominant protein, casein, which constitutes 80% of CM protein, is heat resistant, whereas whey, the remainder of CM protein, is heat labile. Specifically, casein bands via gel electrophoresis have been shown to remain stable after 50 minutes of boiling (203°F), whereas whey protein bands were undetectable after 15 minutes of heating. Bloom and colleagues[11] also found that subjects who reacted to baked milk had stronger IgE binding to casein when compared with subjects who did not react.

In addition to heated food proteins, combination with other ingredients like protein, fats, and sugars can modify allergenicity. Kato and colleagues[13] found that EW mixed with wheat flour and then baked led to the formation of high-molecular-weight complexes with decreased antigenic activity of OVM and little to no IgE binding to OVM. When compared with heated egg/milk products alone, heated egg/milk with wheat has shown decreased IgE reactivity via immunoblot.[11,14] This interaction between wheat and allergic food proteins has been attributed to the formation of a matrix between gluten from the wheat flour and the suspected food protein, thereby decreasing bioavailability and exposure to the immune system.[11,13]

PREDICTABILITY OF ALLERGY TESTING FOR BAKED EGG OR BAKED MILK TOLERANCE VERSUS ALLERGY

Before considering any particular biomarker or cutoff value, it is important to assess a history of clinical tolerance to baked goods when evaluating patients with suspected egg or CM allergy. Most patients who declined a baked egg challenge in one study did so because they were already tolerating baked egg products in their diet (n = 76 of 106).[15] If patients demonstrate a reliable history of tolerance to baked goods, an OFC is not needed; they should be encouraged to continue eating those foods, following the recommendations included in **Boxes 1** and **2**.

Unfortunately, reliable biomarkers for baked egg or baked CM tolerance have yet to be identified. Several studies have attempted to establish particular cutoffs or predictive values using skin prick testing (SPT) and serum sIgE measurements; however,

---

Box 1
Recommendations for dietary introduction of baked egg after passing oral food challenge

Baked Egg Instructions

Your child has passed a physician-supervised OFC to baked egg and is now approved to eat baked/extensively heated egg products at home and should do so on a regular basis.
   Continue to carry your epinephrine autoinjector at all times. If your child has an allergic reaction to baked egg, administer appropriate care and document what your child ate (ingredients, food preparation) and his or her symptoms. Please call our office once your child is stable to evaluate your child's reaction. Avoid eating baked egg until you speak with your allergist.

We recommend that your child eat at least 1 serving of baked egg per day in the following forms:
- Eat homemade baked goods with 1 egg per 1.0 c of flour. All homemade baked products should be baked at 350°F or greater for at least 30 minutes.
- All baked products should be cooked throughout, without soft or soggy areas.
- If your child is not allergic to wheat, wheat flour should be used (do not use gluten-free flours).
- Eat store-bought baked products with egg listed as a minor ingredient. Egg should be listed as the fourth ingredient or lower (not in the top 3) when viewing the list of ingredients.

Continue to STRICTLY AVOID any unbaked egg, including the following:
- Any store-bought baked product with egg listed as the first, second, or third ingredient
- Mayonnaise
- Creamy salad dressings (Caesar, ranch, blue cheese, Thousand Island, and so forth)
- Eggnog
- Meringue or meringue powder
- Ice creams containing eggs
- Hollandaise or béarnaise sauces
- Soufflé
- Quiche
- Deviled foods
- Marshmallow cream
- Angel food cake
- Eclairs, custard, mousse, frosting or whipped desserts containing eggs
- Bavarian cream, fondants, nougats, frosting or icings or other candies containing eggs
- Health drinks or orange Julius drinks made with eggs
- Scrambled eggs or other cooked eggs (hardboiled, scrambled, or poached)
- French toast, waffles, or pancakes (if egg is first or second ingredient)
- Egg noodles
- Foods breaded with egg, like chicken nuggets or other fried foods (unless reheated at ≥350° for >30 minutes)

Box 2
Recommendations for dietary introduction of baked milk after passing the oral food challenge

Baked Milk Instructions

Your child has passed a physician-supervised OFC to baked milk and is now approved to eat baked/extensively heated milk products at home and should do so on a regular basis.
Please continue to carry your epinephrine autoinjector at all times. If your child has an allergic reaction to baked milk, administer appropriate care and document what your child ate (ingredients, food preparation) and his or her symptoms. Please call the physician's office once your child is stable to evaluate your child's reaction. Avoid eating baked milk until you speak with your allergist.

We recommend that your child eat at least 1 serving of baked milk per day in the following forms:
• Eat homemade baked goods containing *no more* than 1.0 c of milk per 1.0 c of flour; all homemade baked products should be cooked at 350°F or greater for at least 30 minutes.
• All baked products should be cooked throughout, without soft or soggy areas.
• If your child is not allergic to wheat, wheat flour should be used (do not use gluten-free flours).
• Eat store-bought baked products with milk listed as a minor ingredient. Milk should be listed as the fourth ingredient (not in the top 3) or lower when viewing the list of ingredients.
• If milk-containing baked goods include waffles or pancakes, these should be prepared as instructed by the food product and need to be thoroughly heated.

Continue to STRICTLY AVOID any unbaked milk or milk-based products including the following:
• Any store-bought baked product with milk listed as the first, second, or third ingredient
• All milk/milk products that are unheated: regular milk, cream, cheese, yogurt, cottage cheese, butter, sour cream, evaporated milk, condensed milk, buttermilk, instant breakfast, or nutritional supplements with milk
• Milk chocolate chips
• Pizza
• Lasagna or raviolis
• Casseroles containing milk or cheese
• Creamed meats or vegetables
• Milk-containing gravy
• Unbaked desserts, such as ice cream, pudding, sherbet, milk chocolates, custard, caramel, and nougat

---

these have yielded varying results. The initial study by Lemon-Mulé and colleagues[16] published in 2008 attempted to define valid clinical predictors of tolerance to baked egg. Those who tolerated baked egg had generally lower, but nonsignificant, EW and OVM sIgE as well as smaller EW SPT. The study showed that only an extremely elevated (>50 kU$_A$/L) sIgE to OVM was highly predictive of a reaction to baked egg but without a 100% likelihood of failing. Notably, some patients who had a very high EW sIgE or large SPT did not undergo OFC. A retrospective study by Bartnikas, and colleagues[17] included home and open in-office OFCs to baked egg; all patients with a negative SPT to EW passed the baked egg OFC, whereas some patients with an undetectable (<0.35 kU$_A$/L) sIgE to OVM and/or EW failed. This study identified a 90% negative predictive value (NPV) for sIgE to EW of 6.00 kU$_A$/L, OVM of 0.35 kU$_A$/L, and EW SPT of 11.00 mm. However, a 90% positive predictive value (PPV) or 90% probability of failing a baked egg OFC could not be calculated; the study concluded that OVM was not superior to EW at diagnosing baked egg tolerance. Similarly, the HealthNuts study, in a subset of their healthy birth cohort, could not establish a 95% PPV for baked egg.[18]

Although the data for baked egg are poor, there are even less data for baked milk. A retrospective review of 35 observed OFCs to baked milk in a standard muffin containing 1.3 g of milk protein found a greater than 90% NPV for casein sIgE at 0.9 kU$_A$/L and CM sIgE at 1.0 kU$_A$/L. As with the baked egg studies, one child failed a baked milk OFC despite having a CM sIgE of less than 0.35 kU$_A$/L.[19] In a larger study (n = 225) analyzing data from children in both prospective and retrospective cohorts, Caubet and colleagues[20] proposed a positive decision point for casein sIgE of 20.2 kU$_A$/L (meaning that at more than this level, patients are unlikely to pass). A small prospective study included 30 milk-allergic children with an SPT to CM of 8 to 14 mm.[21] They performed SPT using a baked milk muffin slurry and found a greater than 90% NPV of 4 mm for the muffin slurry and casein sIgE of 6 kU$_A$/L. All children with a negative muffin SPT passed OFC. Similar to the baked egg studies, a larger SPT to CM and higher sIgE values to CM and casein trended toward a higher likelihood of failing baked milk OFC.

Many providers have attempted to use various sIgE cutoffs for EW, CM, casein, and/or OVM to improve the safety of OFCs or ensure higher pass rates; but unfortunately, there is limited evidence to support specific cutoff values. The poor quality of many of the studies, as discussed elsewhere in this article, and the lack of homogeneity have added to this challenge. A recent systematic review could not recommend any cutoff values for baked milk or baked egg.[22] Given the poor performance of all biomarkers at predicting baked egg or baked milk tolerance, it is reasonable to consider offering an OFC to all patients. Those patients with a mild reaction to CM or egg can be considered for home challenge; or, alternatively, all patients who have not previously tolerated baked goods can be offered an observed, in-office OFC.

ORAL FOOD CHALLENGES TO BAKED EGG AND BAKED MILK

Several studies have demonstrated high pass rates to baked egg and baked milk challenges in egg- and CM-allergic children. In a study performed by Nowak-Wegrzyn and colleagues,[23] 75% (n = 75 of 100) of confirmed CM-allergic children (mean age 7.5 years) tolerated baked CM on observed OFCs, in the form of a baked muffin or cooked waffle, containing 1.3 g CM protein. Muffins were baked at 350°F for 30 minutes in an oven, and waffles were cooked at 500°F for 3 minutes in a waffle maker. Similarly, 80% (n = 126 of 157) of confirmed egg-allergic children (mean age 14.5 months) tolerated a baked egg muffin challenge.[15] Muffins were baked for 30 minutes at 350°F and contained 1.1 g egg protein. In contrast to these studies, Ando and colleagues[24] reported a lower pass rate of 43% (n = 29 of 67) to baked egg in children (median age 34.5 months) with proven egg allergy. In this study, liquid EW was heated to 194°F, freeze dried, and turned into a powder substance. The lower pass rate for heated EW, compared with previous studies, may be attributed to the lower heat temperature and lack of wheat matrix, both of which have been demonstrated to reduce food protein allergenicity. Overall, rates of tolerance to egg and CM in baked goods of roughly 70% to 80% have been duplicated in several studies, despite differing methodologies.[25]

In a multicenter longitudinal study evaluating CM allergy in children aged 3 to 15 months, Wood and colleagues[5] reported that of children with CM allergy, 20.6% (n = 32 of 155) were already ingesting some baked CM products. They also noted CM-allergic children who were tolerating baked CM without a reaction had increased food allergy resolution (relative hazard, 4.1; P<.0001) compared with children who had an adverse reaction to baked CM products (relative hazard, 0.28; P = .72).

The muffin recipes developed by nutrition staff and used for baked egg and baked milk OFCs at National Jewish Health in Denver, Colorado are included in **Boxes 3** and **4**. The baked egg recipe contains approximately 2.2 g of egg protein or one-third of an egg per muffin. Notably, this is double the amount of egg that patients are instructed to eat per serving after passing the OFC. The baked milk recipe contains approximately 1.3 g of milk protein per muffin and is also double the amount recommended per serving. **Box 5** includes recommendations for baked-egg and baked-milk observed OFCs, which includes dosing steps and protein contents. Some providers may wish to take more caution when performing an OFC in certain patients and could consider a more conservative dosing schedule than what is included in **Box 5** (eg, starting with a dose of one thirty-second of a muffin).

SAFETY OF BAKED MILK AND BAKED EGG ORAL FOOD CHALLENGES

Given the lack of predictable markers for heated CM and egg tolerance and the potential for mild to severe food allergic reactions, most children should undergo a

---

Box 3
Baked egg recipe developed at National Jewish Health

Yield: 6 muffins (approximately 2.2 g egg protein or one-third egg per muffin)

Serving size: 1 muffin

Average muffin weight = 73.65 g (−4.45/+3.65 g)

Ingredients

Dry Ingredients
☐ 1.0 c all-purpose flour (or wheat-free substitute)
☐ 0.5 c sugar
☐ 0.25 tsp salt
☐ 1.0 tsp baking powder

Wet Ingredients
☐ 2.0 tbsp milk or milk alternative if your child is allergic to milk (rice, oat, soy, or almond milk)
☐ 2 large eggs
☐ 0.5 tsp vanilla extract
☐ 0.25 c oil (vegetable, corn, olive, or canola oil)
☐ 1.0 c ripe banana or apple sauce

Directions
1. Preheat the oven to 350°F.
2. Line a muffin pan with 6 muffin liners and spray with cooking spray so that the product does not stick to the liner.
3. Mix together the wet ingredients (milk/milk substitute, eggs, vanilla extract, oil, and mashed banana or apple sauce). Set aside.
4. In a separate mixing bowl, mix together the dry ingredients (flour, sugar, salt, and baking powder). Set aside.
5. Add the liquid ingredients to the dry ingredients. Stir until combined. Some small lumps may remain.
6. Divide the batter into the 6 prepared muffin liners (about 0.33 c of batter per muffin). Depending on the size of your muffin tin, you may need to fill the muffin liners all the way to the top.
7. Bake for 20 to 25 minutes or until golden brown and firm to the touch.

Note: Muffins will freeze well. Wrap each muffin tightly in plastic wrap before freezing. Thaw for 24 hours in the refrigerator.

Box 4
Baked milk (egg-free) recipe developed at National Jewish Health

Yield: 6 muffins (approximately 1.3 g milk protein per muffin)

Serving size: 1 muffin

Average muffin weight = 59.13 g (−2.09/+1.87 g)

Ingredients

Dry Ingredients
- ☐ 1.0 c all-purpose flour
- ☐ 2.0 tbsp sugar
- ☐ 0.25 tsp salt
- ☐ 1.0 tsp baking powder

Wet Ingredients
- ☐ 22.5 g (7.8 g protein) dry milk, reconstituted with 4.0 oz of water
- ☐ 1.0 tsp Ener-G egg replacer, beaten in 2.0 tbsp water
- ☐ 2.0 tbsp oil (vegetable, corn, olive, or canola oil)
- ☐ 1.0 c ripe banana or apple sauce

Directions
1. Preheat the oven to 350°F.
2. Line a muffin pan with 6 muffin liners and spray with cooking spray so that the product does not stick to the liner.
3. Mix together the wet ingredients (dry milk, egg replacement, oil, and mashed banana or applesauce). Set aside.
4. In a separate mixing bowl, mix together the dry ingredients (flour, sugar, salt, and baking powder). Set aside.
5. Add the liquid ingredients to the dry ingredients. Stir until combined. Some small lumps may remain.
6. Divide the batter into the 6 prepared muffin liners (about 0.25 c and 1.0 tsp of batter per each muffin). Depending on the size of your muffin tin, you may need to fill the muffin liners all the way to the top.
7. Bake for 30 to 35 minutes or until golden brown and firm to the touch.

Note: Muffins will freeze well. Wrap each muffin tightly in plastic wrap before freezing. Thaw for 24 hours in the refrigerator.

---

physician-supervised OFC before eating these foods at home. Although uncommon, anaphylaxis to baked CM and egg can occur. Out of 100 OFCs to baked egg in children aged 1 to 19 years, with a known egg allergy, 31% experienced an adverse reaction to baked egg.[26] Of these 31 reactions, most were mild, whereas 13% (n = 4) required intramuscular epinephrine for anaphylaxis. During an OFC to heated CM of 100 children with CM allergy, 23% reacted to baked milk.[23] Of those who reacted, 35% (n = 8) experienced anaphylaxis and were treated with intramuscular epinephrine.[23] Among other studies on baked egg and baked CM, the failure rate typically ranges from 15% to 35%, with less than one-third of subjects requiring epinephrine.[25]

TOLERANCE AND ADHERENCE TO DIETS CONTAINING BAKED MILK AND EGG

On successful OFC, regular incorporation of baked egg and baked CM is generally well-tolerated by children. Given the importance of decreased allergenicity via extensive heating and formation of a matrix, it is essential to provide patients and families with clear dietary guidelines of products containing baked CM and baked egg that are safe to eat. In the study by Nowak-Wegrzyn and colleagues,[23] one subject who

evidence is lacking in this area. However, a retrospective study (n = 16) in children without IgE-mediated food allergy found that 73% of patients maintained histologic remission of EoE while eating baked milk (2–3 servings per week) for 6 weeks.[35] The safety of baked egg in patients with EoE is unknown, and caution is recommended with the introduction of baked goods into the diets of patients with EoE.

SUMMARY

CM and hen's egg represent the most common IgE-mediated food allergies in young children, but they are commonly outgrown. Most children with these allergies can tolerate CM or egg in baked form. Given the poor performance of standard allergy sensitization tests for baked egg and baked milk tolerance, most patients with egg or CM allergy should be considered for an OFC to baked goods. Eating baked goods containing egg or CM may hasten the development of tolerance to these foods in unheated forms, and this can be considered a form of oral immunotherapy. Diets containing egg and CM in baked goods are well-tolerated after passing an OFC and can improve the quality of life for families with food allergy. Children with a new diagnosis of egg or CM allergy, but prior tolerance of these foods in baked goods, should be instructed to continue eating the allergenic food in baked form. Further research is needed to confirm the effects of consuming baked goods on the development of tolerance to unheated egg or CM, understand the role for baked cheese, and ultimately develop valid biomarkers of tolerance to baked goods.

REFERENCES

1. Liu AH, Jaramillo R, Sicherer SH, et al. National prevalence and risk factors for food allergy and relationship to asthma: results from the National Health and Nutrition Examination Survey 2005-2006. J Allergy Clin Immunol 2010;126(4): 798–806.e13.
2. Sampson HA, Aceves S, Bock SA, et al. Food allergy: a practice parameter update-2014. J Allergy Clin Immunol 2014;134(5):1016–25.e43.
3. Muraro A, Werfel T, Hoffmann-Sommergruber K, et al. EAACI food allergy and anaphylaxis guidelines: diagnosis and management of food allergy. Allergy 2014;69(8):1008–25.
4. Christie L, Hine RJ, Parker JG, et al. Food allergies in children affect nutrient intake and growth. J Am Diet Assoc 2002;102(11):1648–51.
5. Wood RA, Sicherer SH, Vickery BP, et al. The natural history of milk allergy in an observational cohort. J Allergy Clin Immunol 2013;131(3):805–12.
6. Boyano-Martínez T, García-Ara C, Díaz-Pena JM, et al. Prediction of tolerance on the basis of quantification of egg white-specific IgE antibodies in children with egg allergy. J Allergy Clin Immunol 2002;110(2):304–9.
7. Skripak JM, Matsui EC, Mudd K, et al. The natural history of IgE-mediated cow's milk allergy. J Allergy Clin Immunol 2007;120(5):1172–7.
8. Savage JH, Matsui EC, Skripak JM, et al. The natural history of egg allergy. J Allergy Clin Immunol 2007;120(6):1413–7.
9. Bernhisel-Broadbent J, Dintzis HM, Dintzis RZ, et al. Allergenicity and antigenicity of chicken egg ovomucoid (Gal d III) compared with ovalbumin (Gal d I) in children with egg allergy and in mice. J Allergy Clin Immunol 1994;93(6):1047–59.
10. Nowak-Wegrzyn A, Fiocchi A. Rare, medium, or well done? The effect of heating and food matrix on food protein allergenicity. Curr Opin Allergy Clin Immunol 2009;9(3):234–7.

11. Bloom KA, Huang FR, Bencharitiwong R, et al. Effect of heat treatment on milk and egg proteins allergenicity. Pediatr Allergy Immunol 2014;25(8):740–6.

12. Urisu A, Naruse M, Ahn J, et al. Oral immunotherapy by hypoallergenic heated and ovomucoid-reduced egg white in subjects with hen's egg allergy. J Allergy Clin Immunol 2010;1:AB21.

13. Kato Y, Oozawa E, Matsuda T. Decrease in antigenic and allergenic potentials of ovomucoid by heating in the presence of wheat flour: dependence on wheat variety and intermolecular disulfide bridges. J Agric Food Chem 2001;49(8): 3661–5.

14. Shin M, Lee J, Ahn K, et al. The influence of the presence of wheat flour on the antigenic activities of egg white proteins. Allergy Asthma Immunol Res 2013; 5(1):42–7.

15. Peters RL, Dharmage SC, Gurrin LC, et al. The natural history and clinical predictors of egg allergy in the first 2 years of life: a prospective, population-based cohort study. J Allergy Clin Immunol 2014;133(2):485–91.

16. Lemon-Mulé H, Sampson HA, Sicherer SH, et al. Immunologic changes in children with egg allergy ingesting extensively heated egg. J Allergy Clin Immunol 2008;122(5):977–83.e1.

17. Bartnikas LM, Sheehan WJ, Larabee KS, et al. Ovomucoid is not superior to egg white testing in predicting tolerance to baked egg. J Allergy Clin Immunol Pract 2013;1(4):354–60.

18. Peters RL, Allen KJ, Dharmage SC, et al. Skin prick test responses and allergen-specific IgE levels as predictors of peanut, egg, and sesame allergy in infants. J Allergy Clin Immunol 2013;132(4):874–80.

19. Bartnikas LM, Sheehan WJ, Hoffman EB, et al. Predicting food challenge outcomes for baked milk: role of specific IgE and skin prick testing. Ann Allergy Asthma Immunol 2012;109(5):309–13.e1.

20. Caubet JC, Nowak-Węgrzyn A, Moshier E, et al. Utility of casein-specific IgE levels in predicting reactivity to baked milk. J Allergy Clin Immunol 2013; 131(1):222–4.e1-4.

21. Kwan A, Asper M, Lavi S, et al. Prospective evaluation of testing with baked milk to predict safe ingestion of baked milk in unheated milk-allergic children. Allergy Asthma Clin Immunol 2016;12:54.

22. Calvani M, Arasi S, Bianchi A, et al. Is it possible to make a diagnosis of raw, heated, and baked egg allergy in children using cutoffs? a systematic review. Pediatr Allergy Immunol 2015;26(6):509–21.

23. Nowak-Wegrzyn A, Bloom KA, Sicherer SH, et al. Tolerance to extensively heated milk in children with cow's milk allergy. J Allergy Clin Immunol 2008;122(2):342–7, 347.e1–2.

24. Ando H, Movérare R, Kondo Y, et al. Utility of ovomucoid-specific IgE concentrations in predicting symptomatic egg allergy. J Allergy Clin Immunol 2008;122(3): 583–8.

25. Leonard SA. Baked egg and milk exposure as immunotherapy in food allergy. Curr Allergy Asthma Rep 2016;16(4):32.

26. Lieberman JA, Huang FR, Sampson HA, et al. Outcomes of 100 consecutive open, baked-egg oral food challenges in the allergy office. J Allergy Clin Immunol 2012;129(6):1682–4.

27. Kim JS, Nowak-Węgrzyn A, Sicherer SH, et al. Dietary baked milk accelerates the resolution of cow's milk allergy in children. J Allergy Clin Immunol 2011;128(1): 125–31.e2.

28. Sicherer SH, Wood RA, Vickery BP, et al. The natural history of egg allergy in an observational cohort. J Allergy Clin Immunol 2014;133(2):492–9.
29. Leonard SA, Sampson HA, Sicherer SH, et al. Dietary baked egg accelerates resolution of egg allergy in children. J Allergy Clin Immunol 2012;130(2):473–80.e1.
30. Lambert R, Grimshaw KEC, Ellis B, et al. Evidence that eating baked egg or milk influences egg or milk allergy resolution: a systematic review. Clin Exp Allergy 2017;47(6):829–37.
31. Tomicić S, Norrman G, Fälth-Magnusson K, et al. High levels of IgG4 antibodies to foods during infancy are associated with tolerance to corresponding foods later in life. Pediatr Allergy Immunol 2009;20(1):35–41.
32. Ford RP, Taylor B. Natural history of egg hypersensitivity. Arch Dis Child 1982; 57(9):649–52.
33. Bravin K, Luyt D. Home-based oral immunotherapy with a baked egg protocol. J Investig Allergol Clin Immunol 2016;26(1):61–3.
34. Lucendo AJ, Arias A, Tenias JM. Relation between eosinophilic esophagitis and oral immunotherapy for food allergy: a systematic review with meta-analysis. Ann Allergy Asthma Immunol 2014;113(6):624–9.
35. Leung J, Hundal NV, Katz AJ, et al. Tolerance of baked milk in patients with cow's milk-mediated eosinophilic esophagitis. J Allergy Clin Immunol 2013;132(5): 1215–6.e1.

Interventional Therapies for the Treatment of Food Allergy

Christopher P. Parrish, MD[a], Edwin H. Kim, MD, MS[b],
J. Andrew Bird, MD[c],*

KEYWORDS

- Food allergy treatment • IgE-mediated food allergy • Oral immunotherapy • OIT
- Sublingual immunotherapy • SLIT • Epicutaneous immunotherapy • EPIT

KEY POINTS

- Approved treatment of IgE-mediated food allergy is currently limited to allergen avoidance and emergency treatment with epinephrine on accidental ingestion.
- Oral immunotherapy has shown promise in recent studies. Most patients achieve successful desensitization but adverse effects are common, including gastrointestinal symptoms and anaphylaxis.
- Sublingual immunotherapy and epicutaneous immunotherapy seem to offer improved safety profiles but lower efficacy.

Food allergy is an increasingly common problem, with an estimated prevalence of up to 8% among young children and 3% to 6% of the entire US population.[1–3] In recent decades, prevalence has increased, especially for peanut allergy.[3,4] The natural history of food allergy leads to natural tolerance for some children, but allergies to peanuts and tree nuts usually persist into adulthood.[5] Milk and egg allergy may also persist, especially among those most severely affected.[6,7] Although life-threatening anaphylactic reactions to foods do occur, overall mortality due to food allergy is rare.[8] Evidence is ample, however, that food allergy has a significant impact on

Disclosure Statement: Dr J.A. Bird has received research, travel support, and lecture fees from Aimmune therapeutics and DBV technologies. Dr E.H. Kim has received research, travel support, and honoraria from Aimmune therapeutics and DBV technologies.
[a] Food Allergy Center at Children's Medical Center, 1935 Medical District Drive, Dallas, TX 75235, USA; [b] Division of Rheumatology, Allergy and Immunology, University of North Carolina-Chapel Hill, 3300 Thurston Building, Campus Box 7280, Chapel Hill, NC 27599-7280, USA; [c] Departments of Pediatrics and Internal Medicine, Division of Allergy and Immunology, The University of Texas Southwestern Medical Center, 5323 Harry Hines Boulevard, Dallas, TX 75390-9063, USA
* Corresponding author.
E-mail address: Drew.Bird@UTSouthwestern.edu

Immunol Allergy Clin N Am 38 (2018) 77–88
https://doi.org/10.1016/j.iac.2017.09.006
immunology.theclinics.com
0889-8561/18/© 2017 Elsevier Inc. All rights reserved.

affected individuals and family members, through morbidity and negative effects on quality of life.[9,10] Approved management of food allergy is limited to allergen avoidance and administration of rescue medications, such as antihistamines and self-injectable epinephrine as needed when reactions occur. Together, all these factors illustrate the need for an effective therapy for food allergy.

Although reports of successful oral immunotherapy (OIT) for food allergy date to at least 1908,[11] this approach was never widely adopted. In the 1990s, attempts to desensitize or promote tolerance through subcutaneous immunotherapy did show increased tolerance to oral peanut challenge, but rates of severe reactions were unacceptably high.[12,13] Interest in interventional therapies for food allergies has increased recently, with substantial research efforts undertaken to investigate multiple forms of immunotherapy (oral, sublingual, and epicutaneous). Although the Food and Drug Administration (FDA) has not yet approved any interventional therapy for food allergy, this article reviews the progress to date and discusses future prospects in the search for safe, reliable treatment options for food allergy.

IMMUNOTHERAPY
Oral Immunotherapy

OIT has received more attention and currently has a larger evidence base than sublingual immunotherapy (SLIT) or epicutaneous immunotherapy (EPIT). Protocols vary, but the general approach typically involves 3 phases:

- Initial escalation
- Buildup
- Maintenance

Initial escalation dosing is generally performed in a single day with 6 to 8 increasing doses. Doses usually start at less than 1 mg and increase to several milligrams. In the buildup phase, patients ingest a daily dose of the food allergen, which is increased at regular intervals until reaching the target dose. This dose (typically several hundred milligrams or more) is then continued for the duration of the maintenance phase. An oral food challenge (OFC) at the end of maintenance assesses for desensitization, a temporary state of immune unresponsiveness with an increased threshold of reactivity. For those who are successfully desensitized, an additional OFC may be done after a period of abstinence to assess for sustained unresponsiveness (SU). Many patients are desensitized during OIT, but fewer seem to achieve SU, although this has not been significantly addressed in most published studies.

Peanut oral immunotherapy

Interest in peanut OIT has increased significantly, beginning with case reports of successful peanut OIT published in 2006.[14,15] The first multicenter randomized peanut double-blind placebo-controlled (DBPC) peanut OIT study was reported in 2011.[16] Sixteen of 19 children (age 1–16) in the active treatment arm achieved desensitization, passing a 5000-mg peanut DBPC food challenge (DBPCFC) after 48 weeks OIT with a maintenance dose of 4000-mg peanut protein. The other 3 subjects withdrew due to allergic side effects.

SU after peanut OIT was first reported by Vickery and colleagues[17] in 2014. In this open-label peanut OIT trial, children (age 1–16) were treated for up to 5 years with a peanut OIT maintenance dose of up to 4 g peanut protein per day. Twelve of 24 patients who completed the protocol achieved SU (passed 5 g OFC) 1 month after stopping OIT. Those who passed had lower levels at baseline and at time of challenge of skin prick test (SPT) wheal size, peanut-specific, Ara h 1–specific, and Ara h 2–specific IgE, and peanut-specific IgE/total IgE ratio.

In a study designed primarily to compare peanut OIT to peanut SLIT, only 63% of patients by intention-to-treat analysis in the OIT group (maintenance dose 2000 mg of peanut protein for 12 months) achieved desensitization, with only 27% achieving 4-week SU.[18] Understanding the correct amount of time to measure allergen abstinence to properly assess prolonged SU is still an area of uncertainty, and it is apparent that SU may be lost with continued avoidance. In 1 study, 7 of 20 patients achieved 3-month SU, but only 4 of 20 maintained SU after an additional 3 months.[19] This loss of SU was associated with reversal of epigenetic changes in regulatory T cells.

The results of the Learning Early about Peanut Allergy study suggest early introduction of peanut is effective for secondary prevention of peanut allergy in high-risk infants already sensitized to peanut,[20] which raises the possibility of an early window during which OIT may be more effective. In a randomized, double-blind trial of high-dose versus low dose OIT for 3 years in preschool children (age 9–36 months), 29 of 37 children (78%) overall achieved 4-week SU, with an SU rate of 91% (29 of 32) in per protocol analysis.[21] It remains unclear if the earlier timing of intervention is responsible for the high SU rate or if other factors, such as lower peanut-specific IgE, are more important. Further studies are needed to further evaluate the influence of age on peanut OIT outcomes. There was no significant difference in efficacy or safety between the 3000-mg and 300-mg dose in these young children. Phase III clinical trials of a commercial peanut OIT product (NCT02635776) are ongoing.

Milk oral immunotherapy

The first 2 reported studies of milk OIT showed desensitization rates of 65.5% and 100%, respectively.[22,23] In a pilot study, 6 months of milk OIT allowed 72% of children to tolerate a target dose of 200 mL of cow's milk daily, with 3 additional children able to tolerate 40 mL to 80 mL daily.[24] Multiple subsequent uncontrolled case series showed desensitization for most patients.[25–27] The first randomized controlled trial (RCT) of milk and egg OIT showed desensitization rates of 64% in the OIT group and 35% in the control group, with 2-month SU of 36% in the OIT group.[28] A year later, the first randomized placebo-controlled study of milk OIT was published by Skripak and colleagues,[29] with a median increase in OFC threshold from 40 mg to 5140 mg after 13 weeks OIT with a 500-mg milk protein maintenance dose. Open-label follow-up showed that the maximum dose was successfully escalated to a median of 7000 mg daily (range 1000 mg to 16,000 mg).[30] Thirteen of 15 patients underwent OFC, with 6 tolerating 16,000 mg and 7 reacting at doses from 3000 mg to 16,000 mg.

Keet and colleagues'[31] open-label RCT of milk OIT versus milk SLIT showed superior rates of desensitization with OIT, but 6-week SU was achieved in only 40% by intention-to-treat analysis, with 2 patients losing desensitization after only 1 week of abstinence from therapy. Long-term follow-up of the studies by Skripak and colleagues[29] and Keet and colleagues[31] showed that less than a third fully tolerated milk 3 years to 5 years after completing OIT.[32] Although most studies include daily maintenance doses, no significant difference in efficacy was found between daily and twice-per-week maintenance dosing while allowing other milk products freely in the diet,[33] but this was based on tolerance of maintenance doses, not OFC assessment of desensitization or SU.

Egg oral immunotherapy

Early studies of egg OIT showed desensitization in a majority of patients in small case series.[22,23] Five of 7 (71%) patients passed an 8-g OFC after 24 months' egg OIT with

300-mg egg white protein, but only 2 (29%) achieved 3-month SU.[34] In a follow-up study with individualization of OIT dose (median dose 2400 mg), 6 of 8 (75%) achieved 4-week SU.[35] The first DBPC randomized multicenter study of egg OIT was published in 2012. In children 5 to 11 years of age with a maintenance dose of 2-g egg-white powder daily, 30 of 40 (75%) were desensitized (passed 10-g egg-white powder OFC) at 22 months, but only 11 (27.5%) had SU 6 weeks to 8 weeks later.[36] Long-term follow-up showed that 4-week to 6-week SU increased to 50% (20 of 40) by 4 years.[37] Recent studies have shown SU of 31% to 37% after shorter durations of treatment.[38,39]

Multiple-food Oral Immunotherapy

Although single foods are the target for most OIT trials, as many as 30% of children with food allergy react to multiple foods, and this subset of children tends to have more persistent food allergy.[2] This lower likelihood of natural food allergy resolution increases the desire for effective treatment. A phase 1 pilot study of multiple-food OIT (peanut and up to 4 other foods) showed no significant difference in adverse events (AEs) versus peanut OIT alone.[40] Results were similar with omalizumab pre-treatment and rush OIT to multiple foods.[41] Further studies on multiple-food OIT are needed to clarify its efficacy, risks, and benefits.

Adverse Reactions to Oral Immunotherapy

Although OIT has been shown to effectively desensitize a majority of patients and even produce SU or tolerance in some, concerns remain regarding the safety of OIT. AEs of concern include IgE-mediated cutaneous, respiratory, and multisystem reactions ranging from hives or wheezing to anaphylaxis. A significant subset of subjects experience isolated gastrointestinal (GI) symptoms (abdominal pain, nausea, vomiting, and dysphagia) with eosinophilic esophagitis (EoE) diagnosed in some. The evaluation of the safety of OIT is limited by the relative lack of large studies focused on detailed assessment of safety.

The largest analysis of peanut OIT safety published to date is a retrospective analysis of pooled data from 3 pediatric peanut OIT trials,[16,17,42] which found that 80% of 104 patients experienced mild (85%) to moderate (15%) treatment-related AEs) during OIT.[43] Reactions were experienced by 72% of patients during buildup and 47% during maintenance, with reaction rates of 2.8 per 100 dosing days during buildup and 0.4 per 100 dosing days during maintenance. The vast majority (91% during buildup and 99% during maintenance) of reactions occurred at home. Treatment of the AEs was required by 61% of subjects, representing 22% of all AEs, with 93% of these occurring at home.

Risk Factors for Reactions

Infection, exercise, and pollen allergy have been identified as factors that can lead to decreased reactivity threshold and increased AEs during milk and egg OIT.[28] These augmentation factors were also seen with home dosing during peanut OIT, with sub-optimal control of asthma, menstruation, and dose ingestion on an empty stomach identified as additional factors.[44] Protocol adjustments, such as holding doses while acutely ill, ensuring asthma control, dosing within 2 hours of a meal or snack, and avoiding exercise for at least 2 hours after dosing seem to reduce AEs. Factors associated with reactions during peanut OIT in clinical practice also included exercise after dosing, viral illness, uncontrolled asthma, delay in dosing, and not eating other food with doses.[45] Virkud and colleagues[43] identified comorbid allergic rhinitis as a predictor of AEs, especially reactions during maintenance phase or during peak pollen months. Increased peanut SPT wheal size was associated with a slight overall increase in AEs, which was statistically significant in buildup but not maintenance phase. Asthma was associated with a significantly higher risk of reaction only during maintenance phase. Peanut SPT wheal size was also independently associated with isolated GI symptoms.

Gastrointestinal Reactions and Eosinophilic Esophagitis

GI reactions (abdominal pain, nausea, vomiting, and dysphagia) are common in OIT.[46–49] Although most patients do not undergo endoscopy during OIT, a meta-analysis noted 20 patients from 12 different reports who developed EoE during OIT with milk, peanut, egg, and baked milk, for an estimated prevalence of EoE in OIT of 2.7%.[50] In a clinical practice setting, the reported rate of persistent isolated GI symptoms was 4.5%, with no comment on endoscopic evaluation or EoE,[45] but an earlier abstract by the same group reported 4 cases of EoE in 75 OIT patients.[51] In the large analysis by Virkud and colleagues,[43] 49% of patients experienced GI symptoms, 33% of all AEs included GI symptoms, and 26% of AEs involved isolated GI symptoms. Ten of 13 patients who withdrew from OIT due to persistent OIT-related symptoms did so because of GI symptoms (abdominal pain, emesis, and dysphagia), representing 10% of the overall population and 77% of symptomatic withdrawals. Three of these patients underwent esophagogastroduodenoscopy, and 2 of them had findings consistent with EoE. Peanut SPT wheal size was the only factor significantly associated with isolated GI symptoms (1.8-fold increase in risk for each 5-mm increase in SPT wheal). A single-center analysis of 794 subjects receiving milk, peanut, egg, and sesame OIT found recurrent GI symptoms (3 or more episodes per month of abdominal pain and/or vomiting) in 8.2% (65 patients).[52] These GI symptoms were associated with higher baseline peripheral eosinophil counts, greater increase in eosinophil counts, and higher maximum eosinophil counts, so the investigators termed the association, *OIT-induced gastrointestinal and eosinophilic responses*. Symptoms resolved and absolute eosinophil counts significantly decreased with reduction or cessation of dosing, and symptoms did not recur for 42 of 45 patients who resumed dosing. Only 3 patients underwent endoscopy, with all 3 showing EoE. It remains unclear what proportion of patients with significant GI symptoms during OIT would have EoE on biopsy, because endoscopy may be more likely to be pursued in those with more severe or persistent symptoms.

Anti-IgE therapy has been ineffective in EoE, and the finding that 2 of 27 omalizumab-treated peanut OIT subjects in a recent trial had symptoms consistent with EoE (biopsy proved in 1) suggests that although anti-IgE therapy may improve the overall safety profile of OIT, it may be ineffective in preventing OIT-induced EoE.[53] Although this hints at shared pathophysiology between EoE and OIT-induced GI symptoms, some features of OIT-induced GI symptoms are atypical of EoE, such as lack of male predominance and the ability of many patients to resume and successfully continue desensitization without return of symptoms. It is also unclear whether cases of EoE during OIT represent new-onset EoE triggered by OIT or, alternatively, recognition of preexisting EoE that had not been diagnosed prior to OIT.

Sublingual Immunotherapy

SLIT is an alternative mode of immunotherapy that offers convenience and potentially an improved safety profile. For years, it has been widely accepted in Europe for seasonal allergic rhinitis, and FDA-approved products for treatment of seasonal allergic rhinitis have recently been introduced in the United States. Mechanistic work by Allam and colleagues[54] has suggested involvement of protolerogenic Langerhans cells in the oral mucosa that ultimately leads to the desensitization and potential tolerance-inducing effect. There are far fewer studies on SLIT for the treatment of food allergy than for OIT, and the majority have been published within the last decade. SLIT has been investigated as treatment of allergies to hazelnut, peach, and milk, and although only 3 separate trials have used peanut SLIT, this is the most reported food allergy treated with SLIT.[18,31,55–58] SLIT protocols deliver no more than several milligrams of protein at maintenance whereas OIT protocols build up to a maintenance dose of several hundred milligrams or several grams of protein. SLIT protocols typically use a biweekly buildup phase and a maintenance phase without the initial dose escalation day because of the lower amount of allergen given compared with OIT. Similar to OIT, OFCs after a set period of treatment and after a period of SLIT avoidance have been used to assess desensitization and SU respectively.

In the first double-blind study of peanut SLIT, using a dose of 2 mg of peanut protein daily, Kim and colleagues[57] demonstrated a significant increase in reaction threshold for subjects on peanut SLIT compared with those on placebo (1710 mg vs 85 mg) after 12 months of therapy. Safety was excellent with 12% of doses resulting in symptoms (compared with 9% on placebo) and most symptoms consisting of transient oropharyngeal itching.

In the first multicenter trial of peanut SLIT, Fleischer and colleagues[59] studied the efficacy of peanut SLIT in peanut-allergic teenagers and adults. After 44 weeks, 70% of subjects on peanut SLIT were responders as defined by at least a 10-fold increase in successfully consumed dose (SCD) compared with 15% in the placebo group. The results were more modest, however, than in the single-center Kim and colleagues trial, because the median SCD was 496 mg. Long-term follow-up of this cohort demonstrated 8-week SU in only 11% of subjects and, despite the presumed convenience of SLIT, greater than 50% of subjects withdrew from the study.[58]

Finally, in a study of OIT versus SLIT for peanut allergy, similar to the Consortium of Food Allergy Research results, Narisety and colleagues[18] demonstrated at least a 10-fold increase in reaction threshold in 70% of subjects treated with peanut SLIT for 12 months and a median reaction threshold of 496 mg. In this head-to-head study, it was noteworthy that the change in the threshold of reactivity with peanut SLIT (22-fold) was far less than that seen with peanut OIT (141-fold) although peanut SLIT seemed more tolerable.

Overall, peanut SLIT has shown promise as a safe alternative to OIT, with significant but more modest increases in reaction threshold and corresponding immunologic changes demonstrating modulation of the immune response. Ongoing studies of peanut SLIT hope to broaden our understanding of the therapy by examining the SU effect in more depth (NCT01373242) and investigating its effect in a younger population of 1 to 4 year olds (NCT02304991).

Epicutaneous Immunotherapy

Another approach with a favorable safety profile is to deliver the allergen through the skin. EPIT was first reported for the treatment of allergic asthma in the 1950s by Pautrizel and colleagues,[60] who used drops of allergen extracts on scarified skin.[60] Recently, the development of a new epidermal delivery system (Viaskin, DBV Technologies, Montrouge, France) has allowed for administration of allergens through intact skin. This technology uses a central polyethylene membrane charged with electrostatic forces to create an occlusive chamber on the skin, leading to condensation within the chamber and subsequent solubilization and epicutaneous absorption of allergen through intact skin. The allergen is taken up by dendritic cells in the stratum corneum, internalized, and then transported to regional draining lymph nodes.[61]

Table 1
Food immunotherapy treatment summaries

	Oral Immunotherapy[16-21,49-52]	Sublingual Immunotherapy[57-59]	Epicutaneous Immunotherapy[63]
Maintenance dose	300 mg–4000 mg	~1 mg–~4 mg	50 µg–500 µg
Activity restriction	• Take dose with meal • No activity for ~2 h after ingestion • Withhold with illness	• Do not eat for ~30 min after dosing	• Do not apply to inflamed skin
Observed dosing?	Up-dosing observed	Up-dosing observed	Initiation and periodic follow-up
Adverse effects	Common mild AEs Frequent GI AEs Anaphylaxis possible	Mouth itching most common (mild) Anaphylaxis rare	Localized irritation at site of patch placement Anaphylaxis not reported
Threshold of reactivity modulation among peanut interventional trials	60%–80% desensitized to 5000 mg with 2000 mg to 4000 mg maintenance dose	1760 mg after 1 y (1–11 years old) 996 mg after 68 wk (12–40 years old)	144 mg after 1 y (more effective 4–11 years old, though trial was not powered to specifically study this age group and threshold changes after more than 1 year of therapy have not yet been reported).

20. Du Toit G, Roberts G, Sayre PH, et al. Randomized trial of peanut consumption in infants at risk for peanut allergy. New Engl J Med 2015;372:803–13.
21. Vickery BP, Berglund JP, Burk CM, et al. Early oral immunotherapy in peanut-allergic preschool children is safe and highly effective. J Allergy Clin Immunol 2017;139:173–81.e8.
22. Patriarca G, Nucera E, Roncallo C, et al. Oral desensitizing treatment in food allergy: clinical and immunological results. Aliment Pharmacol Ther 2003;17: 459–65.
23. Patriarca G, Schiavino D, Nucera E, et al. Food allergy in children: results of a standardized protocol for oral desensitization. Hepatogastroenterology 1998; 45:52–8.
24. Meglio P, Bartone E, Plantamura M, et al. A protocol for oral desensitization in children with IgE-mediated cow's milk allergy. Allergy 2004;59:980–7.
25. Zapatero L, Alonso E, Fuentes V, et al. Oral desensitization in children with cow's milk allergy. J Investig Allergol Clin Immunol 2008;18:389–96.
26. Alvaro M, Giner MT, Vazquez M, et al. Specific oral desensitization in children with IgE-mediated cow's milk allergy. Evolution in one year. Eur J Pediatr 2012;171: 1389–95.
27. Sanchez-Garcia S, Rodriguez del Rio P, Escudero C, et al. Efficacy of oral immunotherapy protocol for specific oral tolerance induction in children with cow's milk allergy. Isr Med Assoc J 2012;14:43–7.
28. Staden U, Rolinck-Werninghaus C, Brewe F, et al. Specific oral tolerance induction in food allergy in children: efficacy and clinical patterns of reaction. Allergy 2007;62:1261–9.
29. Skripak JM, Nash SD, Rowley H, et al. A randomized, double-blind, placebo-controlled study of milk oral immunotherapy for cow's milk allergy. J Allergy Clin Immunol 2008;122:1154–60.
30. Narisety SD, Skripak JM, Steele P, et al. Open-label maintenance after milk oral immunotherapy for IgE-mediated cow's milk allergy. J Allergy Clin Immunol 2009;124:610–2.
31. Keet CA, Frischmeyer-Guerrerio PA, Thyagarajan A, et al. The safety and efficacy of sublingual and oral immunotherapy for milk allergy. J Allergy Clin Immunol 2012;129:448–55, 55.e1–5.
32. Keet CA, Seopaul S, Knorr S, et al. Long-term follow-up of oral immunotherapy for cow's milk allergy. J Allergy Clin Immunol 2013;132:737–9.e6.
33. Pajno GB, Caminiti L, Ruggeri P, et al. Oral immunotherapy for cow's milk allergy with a weekly up-dosing regimen: a randomized single-blind controlled study. Ann Allergy Asthma Immunol 2010;105:376–81.
34. Buchanan AD, Green TD, Jones SM, et al. Egg oral immunotherapy in nonanaphylactic children with egg allergy. J Allergy Clin Immunol 2007;119:199–205.
35. Vickery BP, Pons L, Kulis M, et al. Individualized IgE-based dosing of egg oral immunotherapy and the development of tolerance. Ann Allergy Asthma Immunol 2010;105:444–50.
36. Burks AW, Jones SM, Wood RA, et al. Oral immunotherapy for treatment of egg allergy in children. New Engl J Med 2012;367:233–43.
37. Jones SM, Burks AW, Keet C, et al. Long-term treatment with egg oral immunotherapy enhances sustained unresponsiveness that persists after cessation of therapy. J Allergy Clin Immunol 2016;137:1117–27.e1–10.
38. Escudero C, Rodriguez Del Rio P, Sanchez-Garcia S, et al. Early sustained unresponsiveness after short-course egg oral immunotherapy: a randomized controlled study in egg-allergic children. Clin Exp Allergy 2015;45:1833–43.

39. Caminiti L, Pajno GB, Crisafulli G, et al. Oral immunotherapy for egg allergy: a double-blind placebo-controlled study, with postdesensitization follow-up. J Allergy Clin Immunol Pract 2015;3:532–9.
40. Begin P, Winterroth LC, Dominguez T, et al. Safety and feasibility of oral immuno-therapy to multiple allergens for food allergy. Allergy Asthma Clin Immunol 2014; 10:1.
41. Begin P, Dominguez T, Wilson SP, et al. Phase 1 results of safety and tolerability in a rush oral immunotherapy protocol to multiple foods using Omalizumab. Allergy asthma, Clin Immunol 2014;10:7.
42. Jones SM, Pons L, Roberts JL, et al. Clinical efficacy and immune regulation with peanut oral immunotherapy. J Allergy Clin Immunol 2009;124:292–300, e1-97.
43. Virkud YV, Burks AW, Steele PH, et al. Novel baseline predictors of adverse events during oral immunotherapy in children with peanut allergy. J Allergy Clin Immunol 2017;139:882–8.e5.
44. Varshney P, Steele PH, Vickery BP, et al. Adverse reactions during peanut oral immunotherapy home dosing. J Allergy Clin Immunol 2009;124:1351–2.
45. Wasserman RL, Factor JM, Baker JW, et al. Oral immunotherapy for peanut al-lergy: multipractice experience with epinephrine-treated reactions. J Allergy Clin Immunol Pract 2014;2:91–6.
46. Anagnostou K, Clark A, King Y, et al. Efficacy and safety of high-dose peanut oral immunotherapy with factors predicting outcome. Clin Exp Allergy 2011;41: 1273–81.
47. Anagnostou K, Islam S, King Y, et al. Assessing the efficacy of oral immuno-therapy for the desensitisation of peanut allergy in children (STOP II): a phase 2 randomised controlled trial. Lancet 2014;383:1297–304.
48. Blumchen K, Ulbricht H, Staden U, et al. Oral peanut immunotherapy in children with peanut anaphylaxis. J Allergy Clin Immunol 2010;126:83–91.e1.
49. Yu GP, Weldon B, Neale-May S, et al. The safety of peanut oral immunotherapy in peanut-allergic subjects in a single-center trial. Int Arch Allergy Immunol 2012; 159:179–82.
50. Lucendo AJ, Arias A, Tenias JM. Relation between eosinophilic esophagitis and oral immunotherapy for food allergy: a systematic review with meta-analysis. Ann Allergy asthma Immunol 2014;113:624–9.
51. Wasserman RL, Sugerman RW, Mireku-Akomeah N, et al. Peanut oral immuno-therapy (OIT) of food allergy (FA) carries a significant risk of eosinophilic esoph-agitis (EoE). J Allergy Clin Immunol 2011;127:AB28.
52. Goldberg MR, Elizur A, Nachshon L, et al. Oral immunotherapy-induced gastro-intestinal symptoms and peripheral blood eosinophil responses. J Allergy Clin Immunol 2016;139(4):1388–90.e4.
53. MacGinnitie AJ, Rachid R, Gragg H, et al. Omalizumab facilitates rapid oral desensitization for peanut allergy. J Allergy Clin Immunol 2017;139:873–81.e8.
54. Allam JP, Wurtzen PA, Reinartz M, et al. Phl p 5 resorption in human oral mucosa leads to dose-dependent and time-dependent allergen binding by oral mucosal Langerhans cells, attenuates their maturation, and enhances their migratory and TGF-beta1 and IL-10-producing properties. J Allergy Clin Immunol 2010;126: 638–45.e1.
55. Enrique E, Malek T, Pineda F, et al. Sublingual immunotherapy for hazelnut food allergy: a follow-up study. Ann Allergy asthma Immunol 2008;100:283–4.
56. Fernandez-Rivas M, Garrido Fernandez S, Nadal JA, et al. Randomized double-blind, placebo-controlled trial of sublingual immunotherapy with a Pru p 3 quan-tified peach extract. Allergy 2009;64:876–83.

57. Kim EH, Bird JA, Kulis M, et al. Sublingual immunotherapy for peanut allergy: clinical and immunologic evidence of desensitization. J Allergy Clin Immunol 2011; 127:640–6.e1.

58. Burks AW, Wood RA, Jones SM, et al. Sublingual immunotherapy for peanut allergy: Long-term follow-up of a randomized multicenter trial. J Allergy Clin Immunol 2015;135:1240–8.e1-3.

59. Fleischer DM, Burks AW, Vickery BP, et al. Sublingual immunotherapy for peanut allergy: a randomized, double-blind, placebo-controlled multicenter trial. J Allergy Clin Immunol 2013;131:119–27.e1-7.

60. Pautrizel R, Cabanieu G, Bricaud H, et al. Allergenic group specificity & therapeutic consequences in asthma; specific desensitization method by epicutaneous route. Sem Hop 1957;33:1394–403 [in French].

61. Dioszeghy V, Mondoulet L, Dhelft V, et al. Epicutaneous immunotherapy results in rapid allergen uptake by dendritic cells through intact skin and downregulates the allergen-specific response in sensitized mice. J Immunol 2011;186:5629–37.

62. Dupont C, Kalach N, Soulaines P, et al. Cow's milk epicutaneous immunotherapy in children: a pilot trial of safety, acceptability, and impact on allergic reactivity. J Allergy Clin Immunol 2010;125:1165–7.

63. Jones SM, Sicherer SH, Burks AW, et al. Epicutaneous immunotherapy for the treatment of peanut allergy in children and young adults. J Allergy Clin Immunol 2016;139(4):1242–52.e9.

Adjuvant Therapies in Food Immunotherapy

Wenyin Loh, MBBS, MRCPCH[a,b], Mimi Tang, MBBS, PhD[a,c,d],*

KEYWORDS

- Food allergy • Adjuvants • Probiotics • Bacterial adjuvants • Omalizumab
- Interferon gamma

KEY POINTS

- Although oral immunotherapy (OIT) for food allergy is effective at inducing desensitization, it seems to have a limited ability to induce tolerance and is associated with high rates of adverse reactions.
- Use of an adjuvant with food immunotherapy may reduce adverse reactions and/or enhance tolerance induction (also referred to as sustained unresponsiveness).
- Adjuvants like anti–immunoglobulin E monoclonal antibody and interferon-gamma improve tolerability of OIT by reducing adverse reactions, whereas immune response modifiers such as probiotic bacteria or bacterial components may enhance OIT-induced sustained unresponsiveness.

INTRODUCTION

Currently, food allergy management relies on allergen avoidance and emergency treatment of allergic reactions. Although most reactions are managed effectively, fatalities can rarely occur, with an estimated incidence of approximately 3 per million person-years for children aged 0 to 19 years.[1] The constant vigilance required to maintain food allergen avoidance and the potential for life-threatening reactions result in a reduced quality of life.[2] Finding a curative treatment is imperative to improve quality of life and prevent food allergy–related deaths.

M. Tang is a member of Nestle Nutrition Institute Medical Advisory Board Oceania and an employee of and has share options/interest in ProTa Therapeutics. W. Loh has no potential conflicts of interest to disclose.
^a Allergy and Immune Disorders, Murdoch Children's Research Institute, Flemington Road, Parkville, Melbourne, Victoria 3052, Australia; ^b Allergy Service, Department of Paediatrics, KK Women's and Children's Hospital, Bukit Timah Road, Singapore, S558076, Singapore; ^c Department of Paediatrics, University of Melbourne, The Royal Children's Hospital, Flemington Road, Parkville, Melbourne, Victoria 3052, Australia; ^d Allergy and Immunology, The Royal Children's Hospital, Flemington Road, Parkville, Melbourne, Victoria 3052, Australia
* Corresponding author. The Royal Children's Hospital, Flemington Road, Parkville, Melbourne, Victoria 3052, Australia.
E-mail address: mimi.tang@rch.org.au

Immunol Allergy Clin N Am 38 (2018) 89–101
https://doi.org/10.1016/j.iac.2017.09.008
0889-8561/18/© 2017 Elsevier Inc. All rights reserved.

immunology.theclinics.com

Allergen immunotherapy has been successfully applied to treat allergic rhinitis, asthma, and venom anaphylaxis. However, an attempt to use subcutaneous immunotherapy for treatment of peanut allergy in the 1990s resulted in high rates of systemic reactions and the approach was abandoned.[3] Subsequently, alternative routes of delivery, such as oral or sublingual immunotherapy (See Christopher P. Parrish and colleagues' article, "Interventional Therapies for the Treatment of Food Allergy," in this issue.), use of modified allergens (See Melissa L. Robinson and Bruce J. Lanser's article, "The Role of Baked Egg and Milk in the Diets of Allergic Children," in this issue.), and cotreatment with adjuvants to reduce adverse reactions or improve efficacy have been investigated with varying results. This article discusses the use of adjuvants to improve the safety and/or effectiveness of food immunotherapy.

IDENTIFYING AN OPTIMAL OUTCOME: DESENSITIZATION VERSUS SUSTAINED UNRESPONSIVENESS

Potential food allergy treatments can offer 2 possible outcomes: desensitization or tolerance. Desensitization is defined as an increase in the threshold for reaction and requires continued regular allergen exposure.[4] This clinical unresponsiveness is temporary and lasts only while allergen ingestion is maintained. Tolerance is the state of prolonged immune unresponsiveness that persists after withdrawal of the allergen for a period of several weeks or months. There is currently no consensus on the duration of secondary allergen elimination required to accurately identify tolerance. Consequently, the term *sustained unresponsiveness* (SU) has been introduced to describe the state of unresponsiveness after a period of secondary avoidance following food immunotherapy[5] and is the preferred term when describing food immunotherapy trial outcomes.

There is a lack of consensus regarding the ultimate goal of immunotherapy. Desensitization offers the individual protection against accidental ingestion to limited amounts of food allergen, however, they remain allergic to the food allergen; hence, reactions can and do occur, including to previously tolerated doses. In the case of oral immunotherapy (OIT), approximately 65%-75% of desensitized individuals reported frequent and often severe allergic reactions to previously tolerated doses.[6,7] Furthermore, approximately 50% of desensitized individuals were unable to continue regular allergen intake because of adverse reactions.[7] Another limitation of desensitization as a treatment outcome is that protection can be lost over time.[7] It is, therefore, uncertain whether desensitization offers an improvement for individuals with food allergy compared with allergen avoidance. Achieving tolerance or SU would seem to be the preferred treatment outcome following food immunotherapy, as this would theoretically allow consumption of unrestricted amounts of the allergenic food ad libitum without a reaction.

LIMITATIONS OF ORAL IMMUNOTHERAPY AS A POTENTIAL TREATMENT OF FOOD ALLERGY

Cumulative evidence confirms that OIT is effective at inducing desensitization in most peanut, egg, and milk allergic patients[8,9]; however, SU is only achieved in about a third of patients following peanut, egg, or milk OIT.[8] Furthermore, OIT-induced SU seems to be short-lived, with 50% of subjects who achieved SU at 3 months after peanut OIT losing SU by 6 months after treatment.[10,11] Suppression of the allergen-specific immunologic response similarly seems to be transient.[12]

Adverse events with OIT are frequent. Reactions requiring adrenaline occur more frequently than with dietary avoidance.[9] Up to 20% of participants fail to reach the target maintenance OIT dose because of significant gastrointestinal symptoms or anaphylaxis[13,14]; 10% to 30% withdraw from OIT trials because of adverse events,[4] and eosinophilic esophagitis has been reported in up to 10% to 15%.[15,16] Most studies excluded patients with severe food-induced anaphylaxis, so reaction rates may be even higher in unselected food-allergic populations. The limited ability of OIT to induce SU and high rates of adverse reactions highlight the need for novel strategies to enhance tolerance induction and reduce adverse reactions with OIT.

ADJUVANT THERAPIES

One approach to reduce OIT-associated adverse reactions and/or enhance the tolerogenic effects of OIT is the use of an adjuvant together with food immunotherapy. Adjuvants may be selected for their ability to suppress the acute allergic reaction and/or modulate the underlying allergic immune response, respectively.

Inhibition of the Immunoglobulin E–Mediated Allergic Response

Anti-immunoglobulin E monoclonal antibody

Anti-immunoglobulin E (IgE) monoclonal antibody (mAb) was first introduced as an adjunctive therapy to reduce OIT-related allergic reactions. Omalizumab is a humanized recombinant mAb that binds to the CHε3 region of IgE and prevents binding of IgE to FcεRI and FcεRII receptors on mast cells and basophils, thereby preventing mast cell and basophil activation. Omalizumab also downregulates the expression of IgE receptors on mast cells, basophils, and dendritic cells.[17] The addition of omalizumab to immunotherapy in patients with asthma,[18] allergic rhinitis,[19] and venom hypersensitivity[20] reduced the number of adverse events, allowing more rapid dose escalation and higher maintenance doses. These findings provided the rationale for using anti-IgE mAbs with immunotherapy in food allergy.

Both TNX-901, another anti-IgE mAb,[21] and omalizumab[22,23] have been shown to increase the threshold of reactivity in oral food challenges. Omalizumab was first used in combination with OIT in children with milk allergy.[24] Eleven children received omalizumab every 2 to 4 weeks for 9 weeks before starting oral cow's milk desensitization. Omalizumab was discontinued after 16 weeks, and daily oral milk ingestion was continued at home. Nine of the 11 patients passed a double-blind placebo-controlled food challenge (DBPCFC) assessing for desensitization at week 25. In another study, omalizumab was administered for 12 weeks before peanut OIT.[25] Twelve of 13 patients passed a DBPCFC after 32 weeks of OIT, confirming successful desensitization. Although most patients had mild or no reactions, 2 required adrenaline at home for reactions associated with exercise, infection, or nonsteroidal antiinflammatory drug use during the maintenance phase (after omalizumab was discontinued).

Subsequent reports support the effectiveness of omalizumab in facilitating faster attainment of higher maintenance OIT doses with fewer dose-related symptoms (**Table 1**[24–29]). However, Lafuente and colleagues[29] described 3 children who were successfully desensitized with omalizumab-assisted egg OIT and later experienced a recurrence of symptoms 3 to 4 months after stopping omalizumab while still continuing OIT. All 3 subjects presented with gastrointestinal symptoms that resolved once omalizumab was restarted. Therefore, the protective benefit offered by omalizumab may be lost as antibody titers decrease and a longer treatment duration may be required for highly reactive individuals to complete a standard OIT schedule. Patients who have received omalizumab-assisted OIT should be monitored to ensure continued patient safety when the effect of omalizumab has waned.

Table 1
Omalizumab

Author	Study Design Sample Size	Allergen	Duration	Outcome
Nadeau et al,[24] 2011	Phase I n = 11	Milk	16 wk	9 of 11 subjects desensitized
Schneider et al,[25] 2013	Phase I n = 13	Peanut	20 wk	12 of 13 subjects desensitized
Takahasi et al,[26] 2015	Case report n = 1	Milk	12 mo	Passed open food challenge conducted after 2 wk of allergen avoidance after treatment
Wood et al,[27] 2016	DBPC randomized trial Omalizumab + OIT n = 28; OIT n = 29	Milk	28 mo	Desensitization: omalizumab + OIT 88.9% (24 of 28) vs OIT 71.4% (20 of 29) ($P = .18$) SU: omalizumab + OIT 48.1% (13 of 28) vs OIT 35.7% (10 of 29) ($P = .42$)
Begin et al,[28] 2014	Phase I n = 25	Multiple foods	16 wk	22 of 25 subjects desensitized
Lafuente et al,[29] 2014	Case report n = 3	Egg	4–7 mo	3 of 3 subjects desensitized; developed recurrence of symptoms after stopping omalizumab

Abbreviation: DBPC, double-blind placebo-controlled.

Wood and colleagues[27] examined whether adding omalizumab to OIT can increase the rates of OIT-induced desensitization or SU in a double-blind placebo-controlled trial. Fifty-seven subjects with milk allergy were randomized to omalizumab or placebo commenced 4 months before initiation of OIT and discontinued at month 28 when a DBPCFC was performed to assess for desensitization. Those who passed the desensitization DBPCFC continued on OIT for a further 8 weeks, after which OIT was discontinued and a second DBPCFC performed 2 months later to assess for SU. Although omalizumab was associated with fewer adverse reactions to OIT and fewer doses required to achieve the maintenance dose, there was no significant effect on achieving desensitization or 2-month SU.

In summary, omalizumab used as an adjunct to OIT seems to be effective in reducing reactions during OIT dose escalation. However, reactions may resume once omalizumab is discontinued. There is currently no evidence that omalizumab added to OIT can increase the likelihood of OIT-induced desensitization or tolerance. Further studies are required to determine if the initial benefit provided by omalizumab converts to improved long-term outcomes. The high cost of omalizumab is a necessary consideration given that longer periods of maintenance therapy may be required to support highly allergic individuals through a full course of OIT.

Interferon-gamma

The balance of T helper (Th)1 and Th2 responses plays a central role in IgE regulation and the development of allergic disease. Increased production of interferon-gamma (IFN-γ) has been associated with a resolution of food allergy in murine models[30,31] and patients with cow's milk allergy.[32]

Hence, the combined administration of IFN-γ with OIT was evaluated in a small case control study.[33] Twenty-five children with egg, milk, or wheat allergy confirmed by open food challenges were assigned to receive IFN-γ with OIT (n = 10), OIT alone (n = 5), IFN-γ alone (n = 5), or no treatment (n = 5). Subcutaneous recombinant IFN-γ (Intermax Gamma) was administered 10 to 20 minutes before each dose of OIT. Open food challenges were performed after completing treatment and 3 months after treatment cessation. All 10 patients who received IFN-γ with OIT successfully achieved a 3-month SU. Dose-related symptoms were mild and delayed in onset, with skin manifestations changing from acute IgE-mediated symptoms to delayed eczematous reactions. None of the subjects who received either IFN-γ alone or OIT alone were desensitized; all OIT participants failed to complete the OIT protocol and withdrew because of frequent and severe reactions. Combined IFN-γ and OIT was associated with increased food-specific IgE, although the skin prick test wheal size decreased. A subsequent study[34] demonstrated desensitization with a combination IFN-γ and OIT, although the effect on SU was not assessed (**Table 2**).

These preliminary results suggest that IFN-γ administered with OIT may support completion of OIT and the development of SU. However, findings should be interpreted with caution given the small sample size. Larger randomized controlled trials are needed to confirm these effects.

Immune Response Modifiers

There has been growing interest in a class of adjuvants known as immune response modifiers (IRMs). IRMs typically signal through pathogen recognition receptors, including Toll-like receptors (TLRs) on dendritic cells (DCs). DCs are professional antigen-presenting cells that link innate and adaptive immunity and play a crucial role in orchestrating the T-cell response. Certain populations of DCs have tolerogenic

Table 2 Interferon gamma				
Author	Study Design Sample Size	Allergen	Duration	Outcome
Noh & Lee,[33] 2009	Case control IFN-γ + OIT n = 10; OIT n = 5; IFN-γ n = 5; no treatment n = 5	Milk, egg, wheat	Depends on food	Ten of 10 subjects who received IFN-γ + OIT achieved SU. None of the subjects who received OIT alone, IFN-γ alone, or no treatment desensitized or achieved SU.
Noh & Jang,[34] 2014	Case control IFN-γ/dual OIT[a] n = 10; IFN-γ/classic OIT[b] n = 5; OIT n = 5; no treatment n = 5	Milk, egg, wheat, soy	Depends on food	Ten of 10 of subjects who received dual OIT and 5 of 5 subjects who received classic OIT desensitized. None of the subjects who received OIT alone or no treatment desensitized.

[a] Dual OIT consists of a dose of interferon gamma with OIT in the morning and a dose of OIT alone in the evening.
[b] Classic OIT consists of a single daily dose of interferon gamma with OIT.

capacity and actively promote oral tolerance,[35,36] through complex mechanisms that likely involve the induction of peripheral Foxp3+ T-regulatory cells.

Toll-like receptor ligands

TLR agonists are more immunogenic than conventional adjuvants and induce long-lasting T-regulatory and Th1 responses resulting in a shift from IgE to IgG production.[37,38] Their combined administration with immunotherapy has been explored as an approach to enhance the effectiveness of immunotherapy in treatment of airway allergic disease, with the aim of shortening the duration of immunotherapy. Combined administration of monophosphoryl lipid A, an adjuvant derived from bacterial lipopolysaccharide that signals through TLR4, with subcutaneous and sublingual pollen immunotherapy was effective in the treatment of asthma and allergic rhinitis in children and adults[39–41]; a preseasonal ultrashort course of 4 doses repeated annually for 3 years provided a long-lasting benefit for up to 5 years after stopping treatment.[42–44] Similar results were reported for CpG-ragweed pollen antigen Amb a1[45] and CpG-house dust mite[46] immunotherapy for allergic rhinoconjunctivitis.

Animal studies suggest that TLR-agonist approaches may offer similar benefits in food allergy. TLR agonists induced a shift from Th2 to Th1 responses in murine models of peanut allergy.[47,48] CpG/peanut-nanoparticles prevented anaphylaxis to oral peanut challenge, reduced Th2 cytokines, and increased IFN-γ levels in peanut-allergic mice.[49] Further studies in food-allergic patients are warranted.

Modified bacteria expressing allergenic proteins

Bacterial adjuvants have also been explored for enhancing the effectiveness of immunotherapy based on their ability to induce Th1 responses. The concept is to use attenuated bacteria as carriers to deliver engineered recombinant allergens to the host immune system thereby inducing Th1 responses to the expressed allergens. The major peanut allergens (Ara h 1, Ara h 2, Ara h 3) were engineered to disrupt immunodominant IgE-binding sites, and these engineered recombinant allergens were then expressed by heat-killed *Listeria monocytogenes*[50] and *Escherichia coli*.[51] The administration of these genetically modified heat-killed organisms to peanut-allergic mice protected mice from anaphylaxis and resulted in a shift to a Th1 response with decreased allergen-specific IgE levels. These preclinical studies led to a phase I trial of heat/phenol killed *E coli* encapsulated recombinant modified peanut proteins Ara h 1, Ara h 2, and Ara h 3 (EMP-123) in human subjects with peanut allergy and healthy controls.[52] Rectal administration to healthy volunteers showed no adverse effects; however, 5 of 10 peanut-allergic patients failed to complete treatment because of severe adverse reactions, including 2 anaphylactic reactions (**Table 3**). Post hoc analyses of immune markers showed no changes in total IgE, peanut-specific IgE or peanut-specific IgG4. Further studies evaluating alternate routes of administration are planned.

Bacterial S-layers that make up the outermost layer of many bacteria have strong adjuvant properties,[53] making them particularly suitable as antigen carriers in vaccines. Anzengruber and colleagues[54] recently evaluated the use of *Lactobacillus buchneri* S-layer fused to an Ara h 2–derived peptide as a candidate vaccine for peanut OIT. The fusion protein induced Ara h 2–specific blocking IgG in the rabbit model, suggesting another potential allergen peptide-based bacterial carrier vaccine approach.

Combined administration of probiotic bacteria together with food allergen

Probiotic bacteria are defined as live bacteria that provide a beneficial effect when administered in adequate amounts.[55] Probiotic bacteria have a long record of safe oral consumption and are generally regarded as safe by the Food and Drug Administration. The most well-characterized probiotic bacteria include species from the *Lactobacilli* and *Bifidobacteria* genera. The only randomized trial evaluating probiotics for the treatment of food allergy compared a mixture of *Lactobacillus* and *Bifidobacteria* species with placebo in infants with cow's milk allergy. No significant difference in the acquisition of tolerance was demonstrated.[56] Nevertheless, probiotic bacteria have potent immune effects and selected *Lactobacillus* species have been shown to support tolerogenic immune responses, including promoting Th1 cytokine responses with increased production of IFN-γ, T-regulatory responses with increased production of IL-10,[57,58] and allergen-specific IgA responses.[59,60] It was, therefore, considered that combined administration of a tolerogenic probiotic together with food OIT may enhance tolerance induction with OIT.

Tang and colleagues[61] performed a double-blind placebo-controlled randomized trial of probiotic *Lactobacillus rhamnosus* CGMCC 1.3724 and peanut OIT (PPOIT) in 62 children with peanut allergy. Subjects received a fixed dose of probiotic (or placebo) together with peanut OIT (or placebo) once daily for a total of 18 months. SU, determined by DBPCFC conducted 2 to 5 weeks after discontinuation of treatment, was achieved in 82.1% of patients receiving PPOIT compared with 3.6% of those receiving placebo, the highest rate of SU reported for any food immunotherapy treatment evaluated in a randomized controlled study to date. PPOIT also induced high rates of desensitization (90%) and was associated with reduced peanut skin test reactivity, decreased peanut-specific IgE, and increased peanut-specific IgG4 levels. PPOIT was well tolerated with no participants withdrawing because of adverse reactions (6 participants withdrew for reasons unrelated to PPOIT treatment); this is in stark contrast to OIT whereby 10% to 30% of participants withdraw because of adverse reactions. Long-term follow-up of participants 4 years after completing treatment showed long-lasting clinical and immunologic benefit.[62] PPOIT-treated

confirm these findings. Immune-modifying adjuvants that promote TLR responses offer a promising means of enhancing OIT-induced SU. The immune-modifying adjuvant therapies currently under development include genetically engineered bacterial carriers expressing modified food allergens and the coadministration of probiotic bacteria together with OIT. The probiotics *Lactobacillus rhamnosus* CGMCC 1.3724 and ATCC 53103 seem to be particularly effective when combined with OIT, inducing sustained unresposiveness in a high proportion of allergic subjects with milk or peanut allergy. Future studies investigating the use of bacterial adjuvant/OIT in other food allergy conditions will clarify whether this combination therapy represents a platform approach for inducing SU in any food allergy.

REFERENCES

1. Umasunthar T, Leonardi-Bee J, Hodes M, et al. Incidence of fatal food anaphylaxis in people with food allergy: a systematic review and meta-analysis. Clin Exp Allergy 2013;43:1333–41.
2. Sicherer SH, Noone SA, Munoz-Furlong A. The impact of childhood food allergy on quality of life. Ann Allergy Asthma Immunol 2001;87:461–4.
3. Oppenheimer JJ, Nelson HS, Bock SA, et al. Treatment of peanut allergy with rush immunotherapy. J Allergy Clin Immunol 1992;90:256–62.
4. Wood RA. Food allergen immunotherapy: current status and prospect for the future. J Allergy Clin Immunol 2016;137:973–82.
5. Burks AW, Jones SM, Wood RA, et al. Oral immunotherapy for treatment of egg allergy in children. N Engl J Med 2012;367:233–43.
6. Barbi E, Longo G, Berti I, et al. Adverse effects during specific oral tolerance induction: in home phase. Allergol Immunopathol (Madr) 2012;40:41–50.
7. Keet CA, Seopaul S, Knorr S, et al. Long-term follow-up of oral immunotherapy for cow's milk allergy. J Allergy Clin Immunol 2013;132:737–9.
8. Tang MLK, Hsiao K-C. An update on oral immunotherapy for the treatment of food allergy. Paediatr Child Health 2016;26:304–9.
9. Brozek JL, Terracciano L, Hsu J, et al. Oral immunotherapy for IgE-mediated cow's milk allergy: a systematic review and meta-analysis. Clin Exp Allergy 2012;42:363–74.
10. Syed A, Garcia MA, Lyu SC, et al. Peanut oral immunotherapy results in increased antigen-induced regulatory T-cell function and hypomethylation of forkhead box protein 3 (FOXP3). J Allergy Clin Immunol 2014;133:500–10.
11. Berin MC, Mayer L. Can we produce true tolerance in patients with food allergy? J Allergy Clin Immunol 2013;131:14–22.
12. Gorelik M, Narisety SD, Guerrerio AL, et al. Suppression of the immunologic response to peanut during immunotherapy is often transient. J Allergy Clin Immunol 2015;135:1283–92.
13. Anagnostou K, Islam S, King Y, et al. Assessing the efficacy of oral immunotherapy for the desensitisation of peanut allergy in children (STOP II): a phase 2 randomised controlled trial. Lancet 2014;383:1297–304.
14. Pajno GB, Caminiti L, Ruggeri P, et al. Oral immunotherapy for cow's milk allergy with a weekly up-dosing regimen: a randomized single-blind controlled study. Ann Allergy Asthma Immunol 2010;105:376–81.
15. Ridolo E, De Angelis GL, Dall'Aglio P. Eosinophilic esophagitis after specific oral tolerance induction for egg protein. Ann Allergy Asthma Immunol 2011;106:73–4.

16. Sánchez-García S, Rodríguez Del Río P, Escudero C, et al. Possible eosinophilic esophagitis induced by milk oral immunotherapy. J Allergy Clin Immunol 2012; 129:1155–7.
17. Prussin C, Griffith DT, Boesel KM, et al. Omalizumab treatment downregulates dendritic cell FcepsilonRI expression. J Allergy Clin Immunol 2003;112:1147–54.
18. Massanari M, Nelson H, Casale T, et al. Effect of pretreatment with omalizumab on the tolerability of specific immunotherapy in allergic asthma. J Allergy Clin Immunol 2010;125:383–9.
19. Casale TB, Busse WW, Kline JN, et al. Omalizumab pretreatment decreases acute reactions after rush immunotherapy for ragweed-induced seasonal allergic rhinitis. J Allergy Clin Immunol 2006;117:134–40.
20. Galera C, Soohun N, Zankar N, et al. Severe anaphylaxis to bee venom immunotherapy: efficacy of pretreatment and concurrent treatment with omalizumab. J Investig Allergol Clin Immunol 2009;19:225–9.
21. Leung DY, Sampson HA, Yunginger JW, et al. Effect of anti-IgE therapy in patients with peanut allergy. N Engl J Med 2003;348:986–93.
22. Sampson HA, Leung DY, Burks AW, et al. A phase II, randomized, double-blind, parallel-group, placebo-controlled oral food challenge trial of Xolair (omalizumab) in peanut allergy. J Allergy Clin Immunol 2011;127:1309–10.
23. Savage JH, Courneya JP, Sterba PM, et al. Kinetics of mast cell, basophil, and oral food challenge responses in omalizumab-treated adults with peanut allergy. J Allergy Clin Immunol 2012;130:1123–9.
24. Nadeau KC, Schneider LC, Hoyte L, et al. Rapid oral desensitization in combination with omalizumab therapy in patients with cow's milk allergy. J Allergy Clin Immunol 2011;127:1622–4.
25. Schneider LC, Rachid R, LeBovidge J, et al. A pilot study of omalizumab to facilitate rapid oral desensitization in high-risk peanut-allergic patients. J Allergy Clin Immunol 2013;132:1368–74.
26. Takahasi M, Taniuchi S, Soejima K, et al. Successful desensitisation in a boy with severe cow's milk allergy by a combination therapy using omalizumab and rush oral immunotherapy. Allergy Asthma Clin Immunol 2015;11:18.
27. Wood RA, Kim JS, Lindblad R, et al. A randomized, double-blind, placebo-controlled study of omalizumab combined with oral immunotherapy for the treatment of cow's milk allergy. J Allergy Clin Immunol 2016;137:1103–10.
28. Begin P, Dominguez T, Wilson SP, et al. Phase 1 results of safety and tolerability in a rush oral immunotherapy protocol to multiple foods using Omalizumab. Allergy Asthma Clin Immunol 2014;10:7.
29. Lafuente I, Mazon A, Nieto M, et al. Possible recurrence of symptoms after discontinuation of omalizumab in anti-IgE-assisted desensitization to egg. Pediatr Allergy Immunol 2014;25:717–9.
30. Kweon MN, Fujihashi K, VanCott JL, et al. Lack of orally induced systemic unresponsiveness in IFN-gamma knockout mice. J Immunol 1998;160:1687–93.
31. Lee HO, Miller SD, Hurst SD, et al. Interferon gamma induction during oral tolerance reduces T-cell migration to sites of inflammation. Gastroenterology 2000; 119:129–38.
32. Suomalainen H, Soppi E, Laine S, et al. Immunologic disturbances in cow's milk allergy, 2: evidence for defective interferon-gamma generation. Pediatr Allergy Immunol 1993;4:203–7.
33. Noh G, Lee SS. A pilot study of interferon-gamma-induced specific oral tolerance induction (ISOTI) for immunoglobulin E-mediated anaphylactic food allergy. J Interferon Cytokine Res 2009;29:667–75.

34. Noh G, Jang EH. Dual specific oral tolerance induction using interferon gamma for IgE-mediated anaphylactic food allergy and the dissociation of local skin allergy and systemic oral allergy: tolerance or desensitisation? J Investig Allergol Clin Immunol 2014;24:87–97.

35. Worbs T, Bode U, Yan S, et al. Oral tolerance originates in the intestinal immune system and relies on antigen carriage by dendritic cells. J Exp Med 2006;203: 519–27.

36. Ruiter B, Shreffler WG. The role of dendritic cells in food allergy. J Allergy Clin Immunol 2012;129:921–8.

37. Aryan Z, Holgate ST, Radzioch D, et al. A new era of targeting the ancient gatekeepers of the immune system: toll-like agonists in the treatment of allergic rhinitis and asthma. Int Arch Allergy Immunol 2014;164:46–63.

38. Hedayat M, Takeda K, Rezaei N. Prophylactic and therapeutic implications of toll-like receptor ligands. Med Res Rev 2012;32:294–325.

39. Rosewich M, Schulze J, Eickmeier O, et al. Tolerance induction after specific immunotherapy with pollen allergoids adjuvanted by monophosphoryl lipid A in children. Clin Exp Immunol 2010;160:403–10.

40. Drachenberg KJ, Wheeler AW, Stuebner P, et al. A well-tolerated grass pollen-specific allergy vaccine containing a novel adjuvant, monophosphoryl lipid A, reduces allergic symptoms after only four preseasonal injections. Allergy 2001;56: 498–505.

41. Rosewich M, Schulze J, Fischer von Weikersthal-Drachenberg KJ, et al. Ultra-short course immunotherapy in children and adolescents during a 3-yrs post-marketing surveillance study. Pediatr Allergy Immunol 2010;21:185–9.

42. Pfaar O, Barth C, Jaschke C, et al. Sublingual allergen-specific immunotherapy adjuvanted with monophosphoryl lipid A: a phase I/IIa study. Int Arch Allergy Immunol 2011;154:336–44.

43. Musarra A, Bignardi D, Troise C, et al. Long-lasting effect of a monophosphoryl lipid-adjuvanted immunotherapy to parietaria. A controlled field study. Eur Ann Allergy Clin Immunol 2010;42:115–9.

44. Patel P, Holdich T, Fischer von Weikersthal-Drachenberg KJ, et al. Efficacy of a short course of specific immunotherapy in patients with allergic rhinoconjunctivitis to ragweed pollen. J Allergy Clin Immunol 2014;133:121–9.

45. Creticos PS, Schroeder JT, Hamilton RG, et al. Immunotherapy with a ragweed-toll-like receptor 9 agonist vaccine for allergic rhinitis. N Engl J Med 2006;355: 1445–55.

46. Senti G, Johansen P, Haug S, et al. Use of A-type CpG oligodeoxynucleotides as an adjuvant in allergen-specific immunotherapy in humans: a phase I/IIa clinical trial. Clin Exp Allergy 2009;39:562–70.

47. Pochard P, Vickery B, Berin MC, et al. Targeting Toll-like receptors on dendritic cells modifies the T(H)2 response to peanut allergens in vitro. J Allergy Clin Immunol 2010;126:92–7.

48. Zhu FG, Kandimalla ER, Yu D, et al. Oral administration of a synthetic agonist of Toll-like receptor 9 potently modulates peanut-induced allergy in mice. J Allergy Clin Immunol 2007;120:631–7.

49. Srivastava KD, Siefert A, Fahmy T, et al. Investigation of peanut oral immunotherapy with CpG/peanut nanoparticles in a murine model of peanut allergy. J Allergy Clin Immunol 2016;138:536–43.

50. Li XM, Srivastava K, Huleatt JW, et al. Engineered recombinant peanut protein and heat-killed Listeria monocytogenes coadministration protects against peanut-induced anaphylaxis in a murine model. J Immunol 2003;170:3280–95.

51. Li XM, Srivastava K, Grishin A, et al. Persistent protective effect of heat-killed Escherichia coli producing "engineered," recombinant peanut proteins in a murine model of peanut allergy. J Allergy Clin Immunol 2003;112:159–67.
52. Wood RA, Sicherer SH, Burks AW, et al. A phase 1 study of heat/phenol-killed, E. coli-encapsulated, recombinant modified peanut proteins Ara h 1, Ara h 2, and Ara h 3 (EMP-123) for the treatment of peanut allergy. Allergy 2013;68:803–8.
53. Sleytr UB, Schuster B, Egelseer EM, et al. S-layers: principles and applications. FEMS Microbiol Rev 2014;38:823–64.
54. Anzengruber J, Bublin M, Bönisch E, et al. Lactobacillus buchneri S-layer as carrier for an Ara h 2-derived peptide for peanut allergen-specific immunotherapy. Mol Immunol 2017;85:81–8.
55. Food and Agricultural Organization of the United Nations and World Health Organization. Probiotics in food: health and nutritional properties and guidelines for evaluation–FAO food and nutrition paper 85. Food and Agricultural Organization of the United Nations; 2006. Available at: ftp://ftp.fao.org/docrep/fao/009/a0512e/a0512e00.pdf.
56. Hol J, ven Leer EH, Elink Schuurman BE, et al. The acquisition of tolerance toward cow's milk through probiotic supplementation: a randomized controlled trial. J Allergy Clin Immunol 2008;121:1448–54.
57. Mohamadzadeh M, Olson S, Kalina WV, et al. Lactobacilli activate human dendritic cells that skew T cells toward T helper 1 polarization. Proc Natl Acad Sci U S A 2005;102:2880–5.
58. Pessi T, Sutas Y, Hurme M, et al. Interleukin-10 generation in atopic children following oral Lactobacillus rhamnosus GG. Clin Exp Allergy 2000;30:1804–8.
59. Rautava S, Arvilommi H, Isolauri E. Specific probiotics in enhancing maturation of IgA responses in formula-fed infants. Pediatr Res 2006;60:221–4.
60. Isolauri E, Joensuu J, Suomalainen H, et al. Improved immunogenicity of oral D x RRV reassortant rotavirus vaccine by Lactobacillus casei GG. Vaccine 1995;13:310–2.
61. Tang ML, Ponsonby AL, Orsini F, et al. Administration of a probiotic with peanut oral immunotherapy: a randomized trial. J Allergy Clin Immunol 2015;135:737–44.
62. Hsiao K-C, Ponsonby A-L, Axelrad C, et al. Long term effects of a probiotic and peanut oral immunotherapy (PPOIT) treatment on peanut allergic children. J Allergy Clin Immunol 2017;139:AB136.
63. Berni Canani R, Nocerino R, Terrin G, et al. Formula selection for management of children with cow's milk allergy influences the rate of acquisition of tolerance: a prospective multicenter study. J Pediatr 2013;163:771–7.
64. Berni Canani R, Nocerino R, Terrin G, et al. Effect of Lactobacillus GG on tolerance acquisition in infants with cow's milk allergy: a randomized trial. J Allergy Clin Immunol 2012;129:580–2.

Complementary and Alternative Medicine for Treatment of Food Allergy

Xiu-Min Li, MD, MS*

KEYWORDS

- Complementary and alternative medicine • Integrative medicine • Treatment
- Food allergy

KEY POINTS

- The prevalence of food allergy has increased over the past 15 to 20 years. It can be life threatening and there is no US Food and Drug Administration–approved treatment available.
- Allergen avoidance and rescue medication following accidental exposure remain the sole management tools.
- Complementary and alternative medicine (CAM) use is common in the United States. However, research into safety and efficacy for food allergy is limited. Continued scientific research into food allergy herbal formula 2 (FAHF-2), refined methods of formulation, purified compounds, and other modalities are needed to improve knowledge about how they work.
- Traditional Chinese medicine is the main component of CAM in the United States. In addition, acupuncture has been reported to reduce wheal size, skin itching following allergen skin tests, and basophil activation in individuals with atopic dermatitis.
- It is important that conventional doctors, CAM practitioners, and patients' families collaborate to comanage food allergies, improve the medicines, and improve patients' quality of life.

Conflicts of Interest: X.M. Li received research support from the National Center for Complementary and Alternative Medicine (NCCAM)/the National Institutes of Health (NIH), Food Allergy Research and Education (FARE), and Winston Wolkoff Integrative Medicine Fund for Allergies and Wellness; received consultancy fees from FARE and Johnson & Johnson Pharmaceutical Research & Development, LLC; received royalties from UpToDate; received travel expenses from the NCCAM and FARE and Universities; received practice compensation from the Ming Qi Natural Health Care Center/Integrative Health and Acupuncture; and is 42.5% shareholder of Herbs Springs, LLC, which holds the patents on FAHF-2 and B-FAHF-2.
Disclosures: The author received funding support from NIH/NCCAM grants, P01 AT002647-01A1, R01s AT001495-05A1/AT001495-05A2, The Food Allergy Research and Education, The Parker Foundation, The Winston Wolkoff Fund, Mr. Pichugov/Mrs. Sherbakova fund, The Drako family fund, and David Schlesinger fund.
Department of Pediatrics, Division of Allergy and Immunology, Jaffe Food Allergy Institute, Center for Integrative Medicine for Immunology and Wellness, Icahn School of Medicine at Mount Sinai, New York, NY 10029, USA
* Pediatric Allergy and Immunology, The Mount Sinai School of Medicine, 1425 Madison Avenue, Box 1089, 11th Floor, Room 11-23A, New York, NY 10029-6574
E-mail address: xiu-min.li@mssm.edu

INTRODUCTION

Food allergy affects 6% to 8% of American children, and 2% of adults. Prevalence has increased over the past 15 to 20 years. It can be life threatening and there is no US Food and Drug Administration (FDA)–approved treatment available. Allergen avoidance and rescue medication following accidental exposure remain the sole management tools. Complementary and alternative medicine (CAM) use is common in the United States. However, research into safety and efficacy for food allergy is limited. Traditional Chinese medicine (TCM) is the main component of CAM in the United States. The herbal formulas FAHF-1 (food allergy herbal formula-1), FAHF-2 (food allergy herbal formula-2), B-FAHF-2 (butanol purified food allergy herbal formula-2), E-B-FAHF-2 (enhanced B-FAHF-2) (derived from the classic TCM formula Wu Mei Wan) prevent systemic anaphylaxis in murine food allergy models; FAHF-2, and its refined forms B-FAHF-2 and E-B-FAHF-2, are the only TCM food allergy products that have been FDA approved as botanic investigational new drugs (INDs). Phase I clinical studies showed that FAHF-2 is safe, had an immunomodulatory effect on T cells, and suppressed basophil activation. The traditional Japanese herbal medicine kakkonto suppressed allergic diarrhea and decreased the number of mast cells in intestinal mucosa in a murine model. In addition, acupuncture has been reported to reduce wheal size, skin itching following allergen skin tests, and basophil activation in individuals with atopic dermatitis. Studies also showed that probiotics and nutrition are beneficial for prevention or therapy. This article reviews recent advances in CAM for food allergy, focusing on herbal medicine and other CAM modalities, including acupuncture and probiotics.

COMPLEMENTARY AND ALTERNATIVE/INTEGRATIVE MEDICINE USE IN THE TREATMENT OF ALLERGY
Complementary and Alternative Medicine in the United States

CAM is a group of diverse medical and health care systems, practices, and products not considered part of conventional medicine but that are sometimes used with conventional medicine and sometimes in place of it. Integrative medicine combines conventional and CAM treatments for which there is evidence of safety and effectiveness.[1] CAM is popular for wellness and some chronic conditions. In December 2008, the National Center for Complementary and Alternative Medicine (NCCAM) and the National Center for Health Statistics (part of the Centers for Disease Control and Prevention) released new findings on Americans' use of CAM.[2] The survey of 23,393 adults aged 18 years or older and 9417 children aged 17 years and younger found that 38% of adults and 12% of children had used CAM in some form during the 12 months before the survey. They included people of all backgrounds. CAM use among adults is greater among women and those with higher levels of education and income. This finding is consistent with the previous survey.[3] CAM includes natural products such as herbal medicines, vitamins, and probiotics, and mind-body therapy such as acupuncture, acupressure, cupping, and qigong. Among CAM users, 75% also used at least 1 prescription drug. In a 2010 publication, 6 in 10 Americans reported using dietary supplements, and 1 in 6 Americans reported using herbal remedies on a regular basis.[4]

Complementary and Alternative Medicine Use Among Allergy Practices

CAM practices in the treatment of allergy/immunology are increasing too. In 2009, the Complementary and Alternative Practices Committee of the American Academy of Allergy, Asthma, and Immunology (AAAAI) reported findings of a national survey of allergy specialists. This survey focused on the attitudes of academy members toward CAM. It found that 80% of respondents were interested in learning more about

CAM.[5] In 2016,[6] the survey of academy members reported that their patients had used herbal medicines (67.6%), vitamins (61.9%), probiotics (57.7%), fish oil/omega-3 (57.7%), or *Echinacea* (38.0%). Many also used acupuncture (57.1%), yoga (52.1%), prayer (48.6%), meditation (41.4%), relaxation (39.7%), deep breathing (33.3%), massage (48.5%), and spinal manipulation (42.8%). The least used were homeopathy (36.2%), home remedies (25.7%), ayurveda (18.2%), folk care (15.4%), qigong (12.7%), and energy therapy (12.5%). Regarding motivations for CAM, 89.9% noted a desire to use natural products and 75.4% cited recommendations from friends, family, or media, whereas 62.3% were fearful of conventional therapies and 58% thought CAM to be safer. The most common indications for CAM use were allergic rhinitis (76.8%), overall health and well-being (71.0%), asthma (60.9%), eczema (58.0%), food allergy (53.6%), and allergy prevention (42.0%). Use of CAM remedies for food allergy had increased from 2002 (11%)[3] to 2006 (18%).[7] The reasons for the increase are unknown, but it might be caused by the different survey population (practitioners vs patients/families). Additional reasons may include lack of satisfactory conventional treatment of food allergy, increased knowledge about food allergy, experience of CAM modalities, and increased scientific evidence over the past 10 years.

Traditional Chinese Medicine and New Drug Discovery

TCM is defined as a medical system that primarily uses Chinese herbal medicines, acupuncture, and acupressure. TCM has a long history and is part of mainstream medicine in mainland China, Hong Kong, Taiwan, Japan, and Korea, where the costs are normally covered by insurance. Integrative practice and research with Western medicines are well established in these countries. Chinese herbal medicines are used in health care and also are resources for new drug discoveries. In 2015, a Nobel Prize in medicine was given to Dr Tu Youyou, a Chinese medicine pharmacologist, for her work in deriving an antimalaria medicine, *Artemisia annua*, from the Chinese herbal medicine herba artemisiae annuae (Qin Hao). TCM is a major CAM modality in the United States and is beginning to play a role in the health care system as a stand-alone or integrative practice. Unlike Asia, the European Union, and the United Kingdom,[8] in the United States, Chinese herbal medicines are classified as dietary supplements.[9] In 2004, the FDA provided guidance for investigating botanic drug products, including formulas comprising multiple herbal constituents.[10] Although preclinical and clinical studies are limited, several suggest that TCM herbal formulas may have the potential for treating food allergies.[11,12]

New Structure of Integrative Medicine in the Treatment of Allergy in the United States

The public uses both CAM and conventional health care. An NIH/NCCHI survey showed that 75% of CAM users also use prescription drugs.[13] Although most of the natural products are generically safe, others may need to be used under supervision to prevent adverse effects or drug-CAM interactions. Traditional medical schools do not provide education on CAM therapies, but there are several approaches available to begin to integrate CAM and conventional therapies:

1. Many major hospitals in the United States have added integrative clinical programs.
2. Training programs to credential conventional practitioners/physicians for integrative holistic medicine or acupuncture so that the conventional physicians and health providers can directly provide CAM for their patients.

3. Collaborations between CAM and conventional health care providers may create a new structure of integrative and complementary services and treat eczema, asthma, allergic rhinitis, and food allergy, among other ailments.

In summary, CAM use is becoming common among patients with allergy and in allergy practice. It is likely that some allergists/immunologists will manage patients with both conventional and CAM therapies to provide more efficient service, prevent adverse reactions, and prevent conventional compliance failures. Furthermore, training programs and medical schools need to educate future practitioners about CAM therapies and develop guidelines to assist clinicians. The Complementary and Alternative Practices Committee of the AAAAI continues to provide resources such as the Natural Medicines Comprehensive Database (NMCD). The 2016 survey also found that 99% of respondents want a "trustworthy internet accessible resource for checking ingredients, side effects, interactions, and evidence based efficacy data."[6]

Food allergy mechanisms and therapeutic targets

Food allergy is a failure of oral tolerance to normally harmless food proteins. Several mechanisms involved in food allergy development have been suggested based on the studies in humans and in animal models, which are summarized here in 3 phases:

Sensitization phase In genetically predisposed persons, ingestion of food allergen induces predominant helper T cell type 2 (Th2) responses partially caused by inadequate helper T cell type 1 (Th1) and/or T-regulatory cell (T_{reg}) cross-control of Th2 responses. Th2 cytokines such as interleukin (IL)-4 promote B-cell activation, switching to immunoglobulin (Ig) E production.[14–18] These IgE antibodies then bind to the high-affinity Fc epsilon receptor (FcεRI) on basophils and mast cells, and sensitize these effector cells.

Reaction phase In patients with food hypersensitivity, reexposure to the relevant foods triggers degranulation of mast cells/basophils resulting in the release of histamine and other mediators, which provoke symptoms of anaphylaxis.

Persistent phase If there is no further allergen exposure following either phase I and II development, some of the T cells and B cells undergo apoptosis, but others become long-lived memory cells and might be the important driving force for persistent FAs such as peanut allergy (**Fig. 1**).[12]

Therefore, therapeutic interventions should target:

1. Mast cells/basophil activation. Because of the slow dissociation rate of IgE-FcεRI complexes, such allergic effector cells permanently show allergen-specific IgE on their surfaces and immediately respond to allergen challenge by releasing mediators,[19] so inhibiting mast cell activation and inducing mast cell disassociation from IgE would minimize or eliminate clinical reactions.
2. Memory IgE response. Long-lived IgE plasma cells have been shown to migrate to the bone marrow and spleen and reside for prolonged periods of time. Transcription factors, including Xbp1, Blimp 1, Blc-6 and p-STAT6 (Phosphorylated Signal transducer and activator of transcription 6), regulate long-lived plasma cells. Therapies that target long-lived plasma IgE cells may provide a curative therapy for food allergy, particularly for peanut allergy. Note that serum IgE levels do not fully represent cell-bound or memory IgE status, and therefore they do not accurately predict clinical reactions versus tolerance.
3. Epigenetic modulation. DNA methylation is a key epigenetic regulator of cytokine expression in the absence of altered DNA sequences.[20,21] DNA hypomethylation

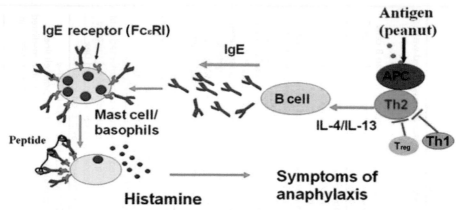

Fig. 1. Food antigens (in this case peanuts) are endocytosed by APC (antigen-presenting cells), allowing T cells to interact with the antigen. B cells are activated via Treg and Th1 cytokines, producing antigen-specific IgE antibodies. These antibodies attach to the FcεRI receptors of mast/basophil cells of the effector organ. Reexposure to the allergen causes cross-linking of IgE antibodies, signaling mast/basophil cells to release histamine and other mediators. The effect is an allergic reaction or, in some cases, anaphylaxis. (*From* Li XM. Treatment of asthma and food allergy with herbal interventions from traditional Chinese medicine. Mt Sinai J Med 2011;78(5):699; with permission.)

activates gene expression and hypermethylation represses it.[20–23] DNA methylation can be modified by diet and environmental factors and is meiotically and mitotically inherited.[20,22,23] Epigenetic regulation of IL-4 and Foxp3 expression is a fundamental mechanism of switching allergic to a tolerogenic immunity.

4. In addition to immediate IgE-mediated anaphylaxis, non–IgE-mediated food allergies include chronic eosinophilic gastrointestinal (GI) disorders and cell-mediated delayed-onset disorders.[24] Tumor necrosis factor alpha (TNF-α), IL-6, and IL-8 may play an important role in non–IgE-mediated GI inflammation, and provide a target for therapy.

CHINESE HERBAL MEDICINE FOR FOOD ALLERGY

FAHF-2 is the first FDA botanic investigational new drug for food allergy. Substantial scientific research has shown that FAHF-2 and refined FAHF-2 products provide long-term protection against anaphylaxis in peanut-allergy and multiple-food-allergy models. Clinical studies showed safety and preliminary beneficial immunomodulatory effects on T cells and basophils (**Table 1**). Studies also began to identify the active compounds from FAHF-2 and other herbal medicines to provide additional vision for developing botanic drugs for treating food allergy and related inflammatory conditions. This article presents the major findings from scientific research, clinical studies, and identification of active compounds that target the major mechanisms of food allergy (antigen-specific IgE, eosinophilic or pro-inflammation).

Food Allergy Herbal Formula 2 Formulation

The herbal product FAHF-2 is based on the classic 10-herb Chinese herbal formula Wu Mei Wan (**Fig. 2**). Our FAHF-2 formulation omits 2 of these herbs, Xi-Xin and Zhi-Fu-Zi, which are potentially toxic if processed improperly,[25] thereby increasing the safety profile of FAHF-2. To enhance its antiallergy and inflammation properties,

Table 1
(continued)

Treatment	Animal Model	Clinical Trails and Human Samples	Mechanisms of Actions
Probiotics	Oral administration of recombinant *Bacillus subtilis* spores expressing CTB-Ara h2 protects against peanut anaphylaxis. Recombinant CTB-Ara h2 spore–treated mice showed significantly reduced symptom scores and plasma histamine levels than sham-treated mice	NA	Oral administration of recombinant spores significantly increased peanut-specific IgA ($P<.01$) and decreased peanut-specific IgE ($P<.05$), but did not affect IgG1 or IgG2at 4 wk after treatment
	NA	Randomized placebo-controlled trial evaluates the novel coadministration of a probiotic and peanut OIT and assesses sustained unresponsiveness in children with peanut allergy	Probiotic and peanut oral immunotherapy is associated with reduced peanut skin prick test responses and peanut-specific IgE levels and increased peanut-specific IgG4 levels
	ImmuBalance, a koji fungus (*Aspergillus oryzae*) and lactic acid fermented soybean product, protects against PN-induced anaphylaxis when administered as a food supplement	NA	Protection was associated with downregulation of Th2 responses. ImmuBalance inhibits plasma histamine and PN-specific IgE levels. Furthermore, IL-4, IL-5, and IL-13 production by PN-stimulated splenocytes in vitro from ImmuBalance-fed mice are markedly reduced, whereas IFN-γ production is moderately increased
	NA	NA	Alive and dead *Lactobacillus rhamnosus* GG decreases TNF-α–induced IL-8 production in Caco-2 cells

Abbreviations: AP-1, activator protein 1; CYP26B1, cytochrome P26B1; Dex, dexamethasone; GATA, GATA binding protein; HDAC-2, Histone Deacetylase 2; LT, long Term; MAPK, mitogen-activated protein kinases; MC, macrophages; mRNA, messenger RNA; NA, not available; NFĸB, nuclear factor kappa-B; OIT, oral immunotherapy; OVA, Ovalbumin; PN, peanut allergy; p-STAT6, Phosphorylated Signal transducer and activator of transcription 6.

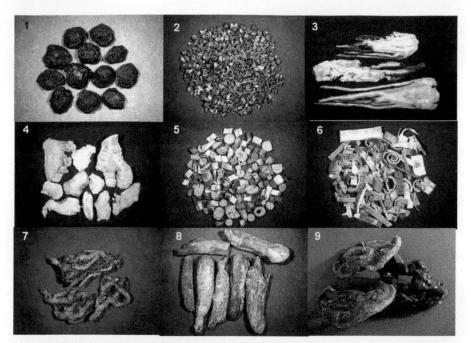

Fig. 2. Herbal constituents of FAHF-2. Based on organoleptic, macroscopic, and microscopic examination, the raw herbal materials used in FAHF-2 were identified as follows: (1) The fruits of *Prunus mume* (Wu Mei), (2) the skin of the fruits of *Zanthoxylum schinifolium* (Chuan-Jiao), (3) roots of *Angelica sinensis* (Dang-Gui), (4) rhizome of *Zingiber officinale* (Gan-Jiang), (5) twigs of *Cinnamomum cassia* (Gui-Zhi), (6) bark of *Phellodendron chinense* (Huang-Bai), (7) rhizome of *Coptis chinensis* (Huang-Lian), (8) roots of *Panax ginseng* (Hong-Shen), and (9) the fruiting body of *Ganoderma lucidum* (Ling-Zhi). Individual herbs are shown.

FAHF-2 also contains Ling-Zhi. Wu Mei Wan and Ling-Zhi, the components of FAHF-2, have long been used in Asia, and are marketed in the United States as dietary supplements. Several studies show the beneficial effect of Wu Mei Wan with or without modification on various diseases, including rash, gastroenteritis, and asthma.[25] No adverse effects were reported in these clinical studies. Ling-Zhi has been found to have antiinflammatory and antiallergy properties[26] and an immunomodulatory effect on Th1 and Th2 responses.[27] Furthermore, Ling-Zhi is also a major component of antiasthma herbal medical interventions (ASHMI), which was shown to be effective in adult patients with moderate-to-severe asthma in a double-blind, placebo-controlled study.[28]

Food Allergy Herbal Formula 2 Effect in Murine Model of Peanut Allergy and Multiple Food Allergies

The authors have established a well-characterized murine model of peanut allergy.[29] In this model, FAHF-2 completely blocked peanut-induced anaphylaxis.[30] The formula has a large safety margin. Mice fed 24 times the effective daily dose showed no signs of toxicity, evidence of abnormal liver and kidney functions, or abnormal complete blood count (CBC) or histology of major organs. In addition, we tested the actions of individual herbs in FAHF-2 and found that the herbs work synergistically and/or additively to produce their therapeutic effects.[31] FAHF-2 produced sustained protection against anaphylaxis, with sustained suppression of IgE/Th2 responses at least 6 months after discontinuing treatment.[32] In addition to modulating B cells and T cells, FAHF-2 directly suppressed basophil and mast cell activation by suppressing IgE-induced FcεRI expression and FcεRI γ messenger RNA subunit expression, contributing to long-term protection.[33] Furthermore, in a murine model of multiple food allergies (peanut, codfish, and egg), similar protection from anaphylaxis was seen when the mice were challenged with the foods.[34]

Moving to Clinical Trials of Food Allergy Herbal Formula 2

The authors have established chemical and manufacturing control data for FAHF-2, including standardization of raw herbs, manufacturing processes, and final product, and safety data testing for pesticides, heavy metals, and microbials according to guidance from the botanic product industry.[35] The authors initially received FDA approval as an IND for acute and chronic safety studies, and then moved to phase II studies.

Phase I trial of food allergy herbal formula 2

The acute phase I study was a randomized, double-blind, placebo-controlled dose-escalation trial to evaluate safety and tolerability of FAHF-2 in subjects aged 12 to 45 years with peanut, tree nut, fish, and/or shellfish allergies. Eighteen subjects received 1 of 3 doses of FAHF-2 or placebo 4, 6, 12 tablets (0.55 mg/tablet) 3 times daily for 7 days. No significant adverse effects were found. All laboratory data, pulmonary function tests, and electrocardiogram data were obtained at pretreatment and posttreatment visits (**Table 2**). Significantly decreased IL-5 levels were found in the active treatment group after 7 days (**Fig. 3**). In vitro studies of peripheral blood mononuclear cells (PBMCs) cultured with FAHF-2 also showed a significant decrease in IL-5 level and an increase in interferon gamma (IFN-γ) and IL-10 levels. Compared with ex vivo data, in vitro data showed greater immunomodulatory effects, which might

Table 2
Summary of laboratory results: acute phase I

	FAHF-2 (N = 12)		Placebo (N = 6)		
	Pretreatment Mean ± SD	Posttreatment Mean ± SD	Pretreatment Mean ± SD	Posttreatment Mean ± SD	Reference Range
Glucose (mg/dL)	78 ± 12	80 ± 21	80 ± 17	69 ± 6	60–120
Sodium (meq/L)	139 ± 2.0	139 ± 1.5	140 ± 2.4	140 ± 1.8	135–145
Potassium (meq/L)	4.1 ± 0.3	4.0 ± 0.3	3.9 ± 0.3	3.9 ± 0.3	3.5–5.0
Chloride (meq/L)	101 ± 2.5	101 ± 2.0	103 ± 1.8	103 ± 2.2	96–108
CO_2 (meq/L)	26 ± 2	22 ± 7	25 ± 1.6	24 ± 1.5	22.0–32.0
Urea (mg/dL)	13 ± 3.5	13 ± 3.4	14 ± 3.2	13 ± 3.0	11.0–25.0
Creatinine (mg/dL)	0.8 ± 0.2	0.8 ± 0.2	0.8 ± 0.1	0.7 ± 0.1	0.4–1.2
SGPT (U/L)	16 ± 4.0	18 ± 7	15 ± 3.3	15 ± 4.8	1.0–53.0
SGOT (U/L)	23 ± 4	23 ± 8	23 ± 4	21 ± 5	1.0–50.0
WBC (x10^3/μL)	6.4 ± 1.4	6 ± 1.1	7.7 ± 1.0	7 ± 1.4	4.5–11.0
Hemoglobin (g/dL)	14.5 ± 1.6	14 ± 1.4	14 ± 0.7	14 ± 0.6	13.9–16.3
Platelet (×1000/μL)	263 ± 44	248 ± 48	299 ± 71	253 ± 40	150–450

Abbreviations: CO_2, carbon dioxide; SGPT, serum glutamic pyruvic transaminase; SGOT, serum glutamic oxaloacetic transaminase; WBC, white blood cell count.

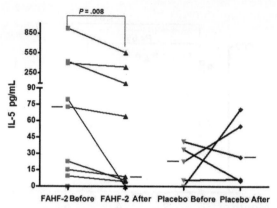

Fig. 3. IL-5 levels of patient peripheral blood mononuclear cells (PBMCs) before and after FAHF-2 treatment ex vivo. Patient PBMCs (40,000 cells) from the phase 1 study separated on a Ficoll gradient were cultured in AIM-V media with media alone, allergen, or phytohemagglutinin (50 μg/mL) for 72 hours at baseline and after a week of treatment with FAHF-2 or placebo. The supernatants were analyzed by enzyme-linked immunosorbent assay (ELISA). Statistical analysis was performed with the Wilcoxon signed rank test. Bars indicate medians of each group (FAHF-2, n = 9; placebo, n = 5). (*Adapted from* Wang J, Patil SP, Yang N, et al. Safety, tolerability, and immunologic effects of a food allergy herbal formula in food allergic individuals: a randomized, double-blinded, placebo-controlled, dose escalation, phase 1 study. Ann Allergy Asthma Immunol 2010;105(1):82; with permission.)

be caused by the direct effect of active compounds on the effector cells.[36] These data showed that FAHF-2 is safe and well tolerated by food-allergic patients and also showed beneficial immunoregulatory effects (favorable for induction of tolerance).

Extended phase I trial of food allergy herbal formula 2
Study subjects were 12 to 45 years of age with documented peanut, tree nut, fish, and/or shellfish allergy (positive skin test and/or IgE). This study was an open-label treatment: 6 tablets 3 times daily for 6 months. Eighteen subjects were enrolled, and 14 completed treatment. The authors measured peripheral blood basophil activation before, during, and after FAHF-2. The results showed it was well tolerated, with no significant adverse effects. All CBC and chemistry panel testing were in the normal ranges. There was a significant reduction (*P*<.05) in basophil CD63 expression in response to ex vivo stimulation after 4 and 6 months of FAHF-2 treatment (**Fig. 4**). There was also a trend toward reduced circulating basophil and eosinophil levels after treatment. It was concluded that FAHF-2 was safe, well tolerated, and had an inhibitory effect on basophils.[37,38]

Phase II clinical trial of food allergy herbal formula 2
This study was a double-blind, placebo-controlled trial. Subjects 12 to 45 years of age with allergy to peanut, tree nut, sesame, fish, or shellfish were recruited. FAHF-2 or placebo treatment was 10 tablets 3 times daily for 6 months. The primary outcome was change in threshold for reaction during oral food challenge before and after treatment. Sixty-eight subjects were enrolled at 3 sites in the United States. Treatment was well tolerated with no serious adverse events. However, the primary efficacy end point was not met, perhaps because of poor drug adherence in 44% of subjects for at least one-third of the study period, because of suboptimal dose and duration, or perhaps because concurrent allergen exposure may be needed because, as indicated in a

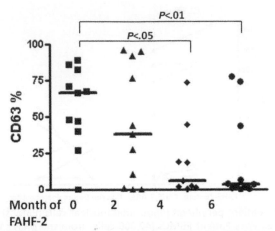

Fig. 4. FAHF-2 suppression of allergen-stimulated basophil activation. Food-allergic subjects treated with FAHF-2. Basophil activation assays (Flow 2 CAST kit) of allergen-stimulated patient blood samples before initiating treatment (0 month) and at 2 consecutive monthly time points during a 6-month clinical phase I study were determined. Decreased percentage of CD63+ cells following 200pg/mL of allergen exposure is shown. P value of <.05 was considered significant (n = 11). (*Adapted from* Patil SP, Wang J, Song Y, et al. Clinical safety of food allergy herbal formula-2 (FAHF-2) and inhibitory effect on basophils from patients with food allergy: extended phase I study. J Allergy Clin Immunol 2011;128(6):1263; with permission.)

preclinical study, mice received periodic food allergen challenges.[35] In vitro immunologic studies of FAHF-2 in the PBMC culture were included in the IND, and the results showed that PBMCs from the same study subjects directly exposed to FAHF-2 and specific allergens showed significant suppression of IL-5 and induction of IL-10 and T_{reg} (**Fig. 5**).[35] Immune cells exposed to a sufficient concentration of FAHF-2 ingredients switched from an allergic to a nonallergic immune phenotype.

Refined formulation: B-FAHF-2 A major drawback of the FAHF-2 formula was the high daily dose. Therefore, a refined FAHF-2 using butanol purification was developed. Butanol purification concentrated active compounds by removing the nonmedicinal compounds, thereby reducing the daily dose. In vitro study using an IgE-producing human myeloma cell line showed that B-FAHF-2 was 9 times more potent than FAHF-2 in suppression of IgE.[39] It was further shown that B-FAHF-2 at approximately one-fifth the dose of FAHF-2 resulted in protection from peanut anaphylaxis in the murine model. The protection was persistent, showing normal body temperature following each challenge, which was associated with sustained suppression of histamine release following challenge, reduction of IgE, increased IgG2a level (**Fig. 6**), and T-cell immunomodulation.[39,40]

B-FAHF-2 Plus Oral Immunotherapy for Concurrent Peanut/Tree Nut Allergy

Srivastava and colleagues[41] recently assessed whether the herbal formula B-FAHF-2 ameliorates peanut/tree nut (PN/TN) oral immunotherapy (OIT) adverse reactions and enhances the persistence of a tolerant state in a murine model. Mice treated with B-FAHF-2 plus OIT experienced significantly fewer and less severe adverse reactions than mice treated with OIT only (P<.01) during the 1-day rush OIT buildup dose phase. Both OIT-only and B-FAHF-2-plus-OIT mice showed significant desensitization

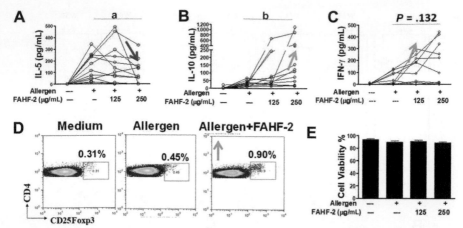

Fig. 5. FAHF-2 suppressed IL-5 and increased IL-10 production in vitro, and increased the number of T_{regs} in human PBMCs. (*A–C*) PBMCs (4 × 10^5) from subjects (n = 12) were obtained at the baseline visit and cultured in AIM-V media alone, with relevant allergen (200 μg/mL), or allergen + FAHF-2 (125 or 250 μg/mL). After a 3-day culture, culture supernatants were harvested and IL-5, IFN-γ, and IL-10 levels were measured by ELISA. (*D*) Numbers of CD4$^+$CD25$^+$FoxP3$^+$ T_{reg} cells were determined by means of flow cytometry. Data were analyzed by using FlowJo software. (*E*) Cell viability was determined by trypan blue dye exclusion. IL-5, IL-10, and IFN-γ production from PBMCs obtained at baseline with or without FAHF-2 in vitro culture (n = 53). Red arrow indicates the inhibitory effects. Green arrows indicate the enhancement effects. [a]P<.05, allergen versus allergen plus FAHF-2; [b]P<.01. (*Adapted from* Wang J, Jones SM, Pongracic JA, et al. Safety, clinical, and immunologic efficacy of a Chinese herbal medicine (food allergy herbal formula-2) for food allergy. J Allergy Clin Immunol 2015;136(4):968; with permission.)

(P<.01 and P<.001 respectively) at 1-week posttherapy challenge, being greater in B-FAHF-2-plus-OIT mice. All sham-treated mice and 91% of OIT-treated mice experienced anaphylaxis, whereas only 21% of mice treated with B-FAHF-2-plus-OIT showed reactions during 5 to 6 weeks of PN and TN challenges. Greater, more persistent protection in B-FAHF-2-plus-OIT mice was associated with significantly lower plasma histamine and IgE levels, increased IFN-γ/IL-4 and IL-10/IL-4 ratios, DNA remethylation at the IL-4 promoter, and demethylation at IFN-γ and Foxp3 promoters. Final challenge symptom scores were inversely correlated with IL-4 DNA methylation levels (P<.0002) and positively correlated with IFN-γ and Foxp3 gene promoter methylation levels (P<.0011) (P<.0165) (**Fig. 7**). B-FAHF-2/OIT may provide an additional OIT option for patients with concurrent peanut/tree nut and other food allergies.[41] These results need to be reproduced in human studies.

Enhanced Refined Formulation: E-B-FAHF-2 and Clinical Study of Triple Therapy

In moving B-FAHF-2 to clinical studies, large-scale butanol extraction of Ling-Zhi proved difficult, so ethyl acetate was used to purify this herb. Ethyl acetate is another safe solvent. It has been used for decaffeination of coffee and tea. The enhanced formula is named E-B-FAHF-2. The FDA approved the study of a combination including E-B-FAHF-2 or placebo (maximum 4 capsules twice daily), multiple OIT to 3 food allergens, and a 4-month course of omalizumab. Primary outcome was sustained unresponsiveness to all 3 food allergens after 2 years of OIT.

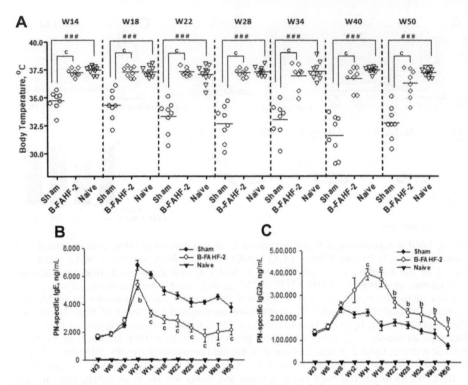

Fig. 6. (*A*) B-FAHF-2 is effective in preventing hypothermia following multiple peanut challenges in vivo. Sham-treated, FAHF-2–treated, or B-FAHF-2–treated mice were challenged immediately completing the first course of treatment (week 14) and challenged again at weeks 18, 22, 28, 34, 40, and 50. The final challenge at week 65 was administered after a second course of B-FAHF-2 treatment. Body temperatures were measured 30 minutes after completion of oral challenge with peanut using a rectal probe. Temperature data for naive mice at weeks 14, 50, and 65 were from challenged mice and at weeks 22 to 40 were from unchallenged mice. Symbols indicate individual mice. Lines are means of each group (n = 8–10) as in **Table 1**. [b] *P*<.01; [c] *P*<.001 versus sham. (*B, C*) B-FAHF-2 treatment mediated persistent reduction in allergen-specific IgE and increase in IgG2a levels. Serum was harvested after blood collection by retro-orbital bleeding at indicated time points. Serum peanut-specific IgE and IgG2a levels were determined by ELISA. Data shown as means ± SEM for each group (n = 8–10) as in **Table 1**. [a] *P*<.05; [b] *P*<.01; [c] *P*<.001 Naïve versus Sham group. ([*B, C*] *Adapted from* Srivastava K, Yang N, Chen Y, et al. Efficacy, safety and immunological actions of butanol-extracted food allergy herbal formula-2 on peanut anaphylaxis. Clin Exp Allergy 2011;41(4):588; with permission.)

Practice-based clinical observational studies

Practice-based evidence studies (real-life studies) can uncover better practices for specific groups of individuals more quickly than randomized controlled trials. This type of study using existing treatment is well suited to determine TCM effects in day-to-day practice. The data generated will be valuable for designing future randomized controlled trials.

Traditional Chinese medicine effect on frequent and severe food anaphylaxis Despite strict avoidance, some severely food-allergic children experience frequent and severe food anaphylaxis (FSFA) triggered by skin contact or inhalation of food proteins.

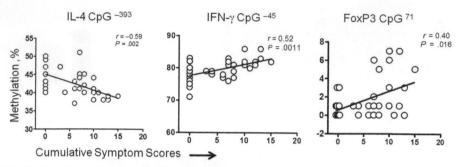

Fig. 7. Correlation between DNA methylation and symptom severity. Correlation between DNA methylation at IL-4, IFN-γ, and Foxp3 gene promoters (shown in **Fig. 6**) and cumulative symptom scores in (shown in **Fig. 4**) following three 50-mg PN, WN (walnut), and CHS (cashew) challenges were analyzed using Spearman correlation.

Recently, Lisann and colleagues[42] published a case report describing successful prevention of FSFA. Three pediatric patients aged 9 to 16 years (one allergic to milk; the others to tree nuts) were analyzed. All experienced numerous reactions (30–400) requiring administration of rescue medications (Epipen use ranging from 5–50 times) and emergency room visits (5–40 times) during the 2 years before starting TCM. These children treated with combined TCM experienced dramatic reductions in or elimination of FSFA, suggesting that the TCM regimen may present a potential treatment option for FSFA. Prospective study of TCM effect on biomarkers associated with clinical protection is underway.

Identification of active compounds for reduction of immunoglobulin E, mast cell activation, and inflammation

FAHF-2 and B-FAHF-2 have shown sustainable suppression of IgE and mast cell/basophil activation, and modulation of cytokine profiles. The authors have begun to identify active compounds from B-FAHF-2 and other resources that modulate IgE, mast cells/basophil activation, eotaxin, and TNF-α production. The major findings are summarized here and in **Table 1**.

Immunoglobulin E Inhibitory Compounds

Two compounds, berberine and limonin, which inhibited IgE production by a human B-cell line, were isolated from *Philodendron chinensis*. Berberine was more potent than limonin in inhibiting IgE production by PBMCs in patients with food allergy. Impressively, the half maximal inhibitory concentration (IC50) value is as low as 0.1962 μg/mL (**Fig. 8**). Berberine suppressed epsilon germline transcript expression by PBMCs, a key mechanism that promotes IgE isotype switching.[39] Furthermore, berberine was shown to be a chemical marker in B-FAHF-2 for quantitatively monitoring its product quality and as a pharmacokinetic marker in animal models.[43] The findings may help develop methodologies to monitor adherence during clinical studies by detecting berberine levels in the peripheral blood and urine samples. The authors recently also found that berberine inhibited Xbp1 and STAT6, the critical transcription factors for developing and maintaining long-lived IgE plasma cells (Yang and colleagues, manuscript in preparation).

Mast cell and basophil activation inhibitory compounds

Because FAHF-2 inhibited mast cell degranulation, the following work has focused on identifying the compounds that directly inhibit activation. B-FAHF-2 was further

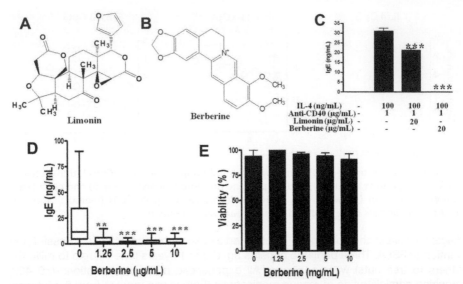

Fig. 8. Chemical structures of compounds (*A*) limonin and (*B*) berberine. (*C*) Effect of limonin and berberine on IgE production by PBMCs from individuals with peanut allergy. PBMCs were isolated and stimulated or not stimulated with IL-4 and anti-CD40 antibody in the presence or absence of limonin and berberine at 20 μg/mL. Ten days later, the supernatants were harvested, and IgE levels were determined by ELISA. (*D*) Berberine dose depended on inhibition of human IgE. (*E*) Cell viability following berberine culture. **P<.01; ***P<.001 versus stimulated, non-treated control group. (*Adapted from* Yang N, Wang J, Liu C, et al. Berberine and limonin suppress IgE production by human B cells and peripheral blood mononuclear cells from food-allergic patients. Ann Allergy Asthma Immunol 2014;113(5):559; with permission.)

fractionated to 4 fractions. Fraction 2 inhibited RBL-2H3 cell and human mast cell degranulation. Three compounds from fraction 2 (berberine, palmatine, and jatrorrhizine) were identified and showed inhibition of RBL-2H3 cell degranulation via suppressing spleen tyrosine kinase (Syk) phosphorylation.[33] These compounds may have value for food allergy and other mast cell disorders.

Eotaxin inhibitor

C-C motif chemokine ligand 11 (Eotaxin/CCL-11) is a major chemoattractant that contributes to eosinophilic inflammation in many chronic conditions. Glucocorticoids inhibit inflammation, but long-time exposure may cause paradoxic adverse effects by augmenting eotaxin/CCL-11 production.[44] Five flavonoids from *Glycyrrhiza uralensis* were isolated and identified, and 7,4′-dihydroxyflavone (7,4′-DHF) was the most potent.[45] It also inhibited Th2 memory cell IL-4, IL-5, and IL-13 production by inhibition of GATA3 (*GATA binding protein 3*) expression.[46] Most importantly, in contrast with short-time culture, dexamethasone (DEX) long-term culture increased constitutively, and IL-4/TNF-α stimulated eotaxin/CCL11 production by human lung fibroblast-1 cells. This adverse effect was abrogated by 7,4′-DHF coculture via modulation of DEX-enhanced p-STAT6 and impaired HDAC2 expression.[47] Studies are underway to test this compound on other types of eosinophilic inflammation, such as eosinophilic esophagitis.

Cytokine modulator

To characterize the active compounds that contribute to the immunomodulatory effects on T cells, the authors isolated 16 triterpenes from *Ganoderma lucidum*, the herbal constituent in both B-FAHF-2 and ASHMI. Ganoderic C1 and ganoderic beta (GAβ) were the most potent suppressors of TNF-α production by a macrophage cell line and by PBMCs from patients with allergies or Crohn disease. This effect was mediated by down-regulation of nuclear factor kappa-B (NF-κB), MAPK (mitogen-activated protein kinases) and AP-1 (activator protein 1).[48,49] A more recent study showed that GAβ not only suppresses proinflammatory cytokines such as TNF-α and IL-6 but also increased IL-12 and IL-10 production by a macrophage cell line (RAW 264.7.).[50] These compounds may be applicable in other allergic conditions related to non–IgE-mediated or IgE-mediated inflammation. Studies are underway to test this hypothesis.

JAPANESE HERBAL MEDICINE FOR FOOD ALLERGY

Japanese herbal medicine was derived from Chinese herbal medicine about 800 years ago, and further developed in Japan. Dr Kadowaki's laboratory has published several studies about the herbal formula kakkonto for food allergy. Using an OVA-induced intestinal food-allergic model, oral kakkonto was shown to significantly suppress allergic diarrhea and myeloperoxidase activity, associated with immune modulation on Th1, Th2, and T_{regs}.[51,52] Kakkonto did not significantly affect OVA-specific IgE. Recently, kakkonto also showed beneficial effects on OIT by enhancing OVA OIT effect on Th2 inhibition and T_{reg} enhancement in the OVA interstitial food allergy model.[53] Kakkonto showed protective effects in an egg-allergic model. Inhibition of mast cells rather than IgE and induction of T_{reg} may be the key mechanisms, and may have a potential for intestinal food allergy.

ACUPUNCTURE INHIBITION OF BASOPHIL HISTAMINE RELEASE

Although there have been no direct publications on acupuncture for food allergy, a study evaluated acupuncture and antihistamine itch therapy (cetirizine) on type I hypersensitivity itch and skin reaction in AD (allergic dermatitis) using a patient-blinded and examiner-blinded, randomized, placebo-controlled, crossover trial. Allergen-induced itch was evaluated in 20 patients. There was no significant difference between acupuncture and cetirizine control ($P>.1$), and both therapies were significantly superior to their respective placebo interventions ($P<.05$).[54] This finding is consistent with a previous study.[55] In a pilot trial, Pfab and colleagues[56] showed that mean itch was significantly lower in the acupuncture group than in the control group, which was associated with reduced CD63-positive basophil levels regarding stimulation with house dust mite and grass pollens. Because basophil activation and histamine release are also involved in food allergy reactions, acupuncture may have a potential for treating food allergy. In addition, more than one-third of patients with eczema were associated with food allergy,[57,58] and acupuncture may be beneficial for multiple allergic conditions, requiring further clinical studies.

PROBIOTICS FOR TREATING FOOD ALLERGY

Probiotics use in the United States is common. However, the publications reporting the therapeutic role of probiotics in food allergy are limited. A study performed a double-blind, placebo-controlled, randomized trial of the probiotic *Lactobacillus rhamnosus* CGMCC 1.3724 and peanut OIT (probiotic and peanut OIT [PPOIT]) in children (1–10 years old) with peanut allergy.[59] The primary outcome was induction of sustained unresponsiveness 2 to 5 weeks after discontinuation of treatment (referred to as possible sustained unresponsiveness). Possible sustained unresponsiveness was achieved in 82.1% receiving PPOIT and 3.6% receiving placebo ($P<.001$).

However, adverse effects of PPOIT-treated participants were common. This study provided a promising approach using combined therapy with probiotics and peanut OIT for peanut allergy. Further work is required to clarify the relative contributions of probiotics versus OIT because the study did not include probiotics or OIT alone.

Zhang and colleagues[60] showed that a Japanese fermented product ImmuBalance, a koji fungus (*Aspergillus oryzae*), and lactic acid fermented soybean product, reduced peanut hypersensitivity in a murine model, which was associated with an immunomodulatory effect on IL-4, IL-5, and IL-13. Zhou and colleagues[61] showed that the recombinant probiotic *Bacillus subtilis* spores with surface expression of Ara h2 reduced peanut-induced anaphylaxis in mice. Further study showed that this engineered probiotic product significantly increased IL-10 by B cells (Zhou and colleagues, manuscript in preparation). In addition, a recent study showed that alive and dead *Lactobacillus rhamnosus* GG decrease TNF-α–induced IL-8 production in Caco-2 cells by affecting the NFκB/IκB (nuclear factor of kappa light polypeptide gene enhancer in B-cells inhibitor) pathway.[62] Because TNF-α and IL-8 have been involved in non–IgE-mediated food allergies, some of the probiotics may be helpful to ameliorate GI inflammation.

FUTURE CONSIDERATIONS AND SUMMARY

The diversity of CAM used in the United States provides a wealth of scientific questions and clinical opportunity to investigate effective treatment modalities for food allergy. The advantage of this type of research is that there is plenty of human-use experience. The disadvantage is that there is limited scientific information available. Continued scientific research into FAHF-2, refined versions of formulations, purified compounds, and other modalities are needed to advance and to fill the gap of knowledge about how they may work. Clinical studies are major undertakings in terms of timing and cost but are necessary to provide evidence-based efficacy with the goal of developing FDA-approved botanic medicines and other treatment technologies. According to the AAAAI survey of the academy members, most allergists are willing to learn more about CAM, particularly natural products. It is also important that conventional doctors, CAM practitioners, and patients' families collaborate to comanage food allergies and improve the patients' quality of life and medicine.

(*From* Srivastava KD, Song Y, Yang N, et al. B-FAHF-2 plus oral immunotherapy (OIT) is safer and more effective than OIT alone in a murine model of concurrent peanut/tree nut allergy. Clin Exp Allergy 2017;47(8):1046; with permission.)

ACKNOWLEDGMENTS

The author would like to express my great appreciation to Changda Liu PhD, Henry Ehrlich BA, and Kamal Srivastava PhD for their help with the article preparation. The author also wishes to thank the clinical and basic research team for their critical contribution to the research. The author also thanks Dr Hugh Sampson for his continued support and mentorship. The author gives special thanks to Susan Weissman and Selena Bluntzer and many families for their inspiration to continue our research to find the cure for food allergy.

REFERENCES

1. Barnes PM, Bloom B, Nahin R. CDC National Health Statistics Report #12. Complementary and alternative medicine use among adults and children; 2008. Available at: https://nccih.nih.gov/research/statistics/2007/camsurvey_fs1.htm. Accessed October 25, 2017.

2. Complementary and Alternative Medicine. National Center for Complementary and Alternative Medicine (NCCAM). Available at: https://www.nih.gov/about-nih/what-we-do/nih-almanac/national-center-complementary-integrative-health-nccih. Accessed October 25, 2017.
3. Schäfer T, Riehle A, Wichmann HE, et al. Alternative medicine in allergies - prevalence, patterns of use, and costs. Allergy 2002;57:694–700.
4. Gershwin ME, Borchers AT, Keen CL, et al. Public safety and dietary supplementation. Ann N Y Acad Sci 2010;1190:104–17.
5. Engler RJ, Silvers WS, Bielory L. Complementary and alternative medicine education: need for expanded educational resources for American Academy of Allergy, Asthma & Immunology members. J Allergy Clin Immunol 2009;123:511–2.
6. Land MH, Wang J. Complementary and alternative medicine use among allergy practices: results of a nationwide survey of allergists. J Allergy Clin Immunol Pract 2017. [Epub ahead of print].
7. Ko J, Lee JI, Muñoz-Furlong A, et al. Use of complementary and alternative medicine by food-allergic patients. Ann Allergy Asthma Immunol 2006;97:365–9.
8. Medicines, medical devices and blood regulation and safety. Herbal and homeopathic medicines. Available at: https://www.gov.uk/topic/medicines-medical-devices-blood/herbal-homeopathic-medicines. Accessed October 25, 2017.
9. Dietary Supplement Health and Education Act of 1994 Public-Law 103-417-103rd Congress1994. Available at: https://ods.od.nih.gov/About/DSHEA_Wording.aspx. Accessed October 25, 2017.
10. The US Food and Drug Administration (FDA), Center for Drug Evaluation and Research. Guidance for Industry Botanical Drug Products. Revised ed. 2004.2004. Available at: https://www.fda.gov/Drugs/DevelopmentApprovalProcess/HowDrugsareDevelopedandApproved/ApprovalApplications/NewDrugApplicationNDA/BotanicalDrugReview/default.htm. Accessed October 25, 2017.
11. Wisniewski JA, Li XM. Alternative and complementary treatment for food allergy. Immunol Allergy Clin North Am 2012;32:135–50.
12. Li XM. Treatment of asthma and food allergy with herbal interventions from Traditional Chinese Medicine. Mt Sinai J Med 2011;78:697–716.
13. NCCAM. Complementary and Alternative Medicine. Available at: https://www.nlm.nih.gov/tsd/acquisitions/cdm/subjects24.html. Accessed October 25, 2017.
14. Cardoso CR, Provinciatto PR, Godoi DF, et al. IL-4 regulates susceptibility to intestinal inflammation in murine food allergy. Am J Physiol Gastrointest Liver Physiol 2009;296:G593–600.
15. Dang TD, Allen KJ, J Martino D, et al. Food-allergic infants have impaired regulatory T-cell responses following in vivo allergen exposure. Pediatr Allergy Immunol 2016;27:35–43.
16. Johnston LK, Chien KB, Bryce PJ. The immunology of food allergy. J Immunol 2014;192:2529–34.
17. Pelz BJ, Bryce PJ. Pathophysiology of food allergy. Pediatr Clin North Am 2015;62:1363–75.
18. Oettgen HC, Burton OT. IgE receptor signaling in food allergy pathogenesis. Curr Opin Immunol 2015;36:109–14.
19. Eggel A, Baravalle G, Hobi G, et al. Accelerated dissociation of IgE-FcepsilonRI complexes by disruptive inhibitors actively desensitizes allergic effector cells. J Allergy Clin Immunol 2014;133:1709–19.e8.
20. Wilson CB, Rowell E, Sekimata M. Epigenetic control of T-helper-cell differentiation. Nat Rev Immunol 2009;9:91–105.

54. Pfab F, Huss-Marp J, Gatti A, et al. Influence of acupuncture on type I hypersensitivity itch and the wheal and flare response in adults with atopic eczema - a blinded, randomized, placebo-controlled, crossover trial. Allergy 2010;65: 903–10.
55. Pfab F, Kirchner MT, Huss-Marp J, et al. Acupuncture compared with oral antihistamine for type I hypersensitivity itch and skin response in adults with atopic dermatitis: a patient- and examiner-blinded, randomized, placebo-controlled, crossover trial. Allergy 2012;67:566–73.
56. Pfab F, Athanasiadis GI, Huss-Marp J, et al. Effect of acupuncture on allergen-induced basophil activation in patients with atopic eczema: a pilot trial. J Altern Complement Med 2011;17:309–14.
57. Eigenmann PA, Sicherer SH, Borkowski TA, et al. Prevalence of IgE-mediated food allergy among children with atopic dermatitis. Pediatrics 1998;101:E8.
58. Bergmann MM, Caubet JC, Boguniewicz M, et al. Evaluation of food allergy in patients with atopic dermatitis. J Allergy Clin Immunol Pract 2013;1:22–8.
59. Tang ML, Ponsonby AL, Orsini F, et al. Administration of a probiotic with peanut oral immunotherapy: a randomized trial. J Allergy Clin Immunol 2015;135: 737–44.e8.
60. Zhang T, Pan W, Takebe M, et al. Therapeutic effects of a fermented soy product on peanut hypersensitivity is associated with modulation of T-helper type 1 and T-helper type 2 responses. Clin Exp Allergy 2008;38:1808–18.
61. Zhou Z, Song Y, Mao C, et al. Recombinant probiotic Bacillus subtilis spores with surface expression of Ara h2 reduce peanut-induced anaphylaxis in mice. J Allergy Clin Immunol 2015;135:AB29.
62. Zhang L, Li N, Caicedo R, et al. Alive and dead Lactobacillus rhamnosus GG decrease tumor necrosis factor-alpha-induced interleukin-8 production in Caco-2 cells. J Nutr 2005;135:1752–6.

Diagnosis and Management of Eosinophilic Esophagitis

Jeffrey M. Wilson, MD, PhD[a], Emily C. McGowan, MD[a,b],*

KEYWORDS

- Eosinophilic esophagitis • Food allergy • Elimination diet • IgG4
- Swallowed steroids

KEY POINTS

- Eosinophilic esophagitis is a chronic inflammatory disease that is commonly food triggered.
- The mainstays of therapy involve the use of proton pump inhibitors, elimination of relevant food triggers, serial esophageal dilations, and topical steroids.
- Contemporary diagnosis and management relies on repeat endoscopy; however, emerging insights hold promise for the development of noninvasive approaches for disease monitoring and novel immune-modulating therapies.

INTRODUCTION

Eosinophilic esophagitis (EoE) is a chronic, local, immune-mediated esophageal disease, characterized clinically by symptoms related to esophageal dysfunction and histologically by eosinophil-predominant inflammation.[1] EoE was first defined as a clinicopathologic syndrome in the 1990s,[2,3] and since this time, it has become an increasingly appreciated chronic inflammatory disease. EoE is now estimated to affect 10 to 50 in 100,000 children and adults in the United States, Canada, Europe, and Australia, and like other allergic conditions, the incidence seems to be increasing.[4–9] Although the underlying pathophysiology of EoE remains unknown, it seems to be due to non–immunoglobulin E (IgE)-mediated allergic inflammation to allergens, which have been shown to be predominantly food in both children and adults.[10,11] In this review, we discuss recent advances as they pertain to the diagnosis and management of EoE.

Disclosure Statement: The authors have nothing to disclose.
[a] Division of Allergy and Immunology, Department of Medicine, University of Virginia, PO Box 801355, Charlottesville, VA 22908, USA; [b] Division of Allergy and Clinical Immunology, Department of Medicine, Johns Hopkins University School of Medicine, 501 Hopkins Bayview Circle, Baltimore, MD 21224, USA
* Corresponding author. Division of Allergy and Immunology, Department of Medicine, University of Virginia, PO Box 801355, Charlottesville, VA 22908.
E-mail address: ekc5v@virginia.edu

Immunol Allergy Clin N Am 38 (2018) 125–139
https://doi.org/10.1016/j.iac.2017.09.010
0889-8561/18/© 2017 Elsevier Inc. All rights reserved.

immunology.theclinics.com

SYMPTOMS

The presentation of EoE is not uniform across all ages. Young children and toddlers typically present with nausea, vomiting, feeding difficulties, abdominal pain, and failure to thrive.[12,13] In contrast, teenagers and adults with EoE tend to present with dysphagia, esophageal dysmotility, refractory reflux, or other sequelae related to esophageal remodeling, such as food impaction.[14–17]

In addition to the symptoms directly related to EoE, there is a clear association of EoE with other atopic diseases, such as allergic rhinitis, asthma, atopic dermatitis, and IgE-mediated immediate food allergy.[18,19] Recent reports indicate that EoE is also more common in individuals with inflammatory and autoimmune diseases, such as chronic rhinosinusitis, ulcerative colitis, multiple sclerosis, and systemic sclerosis.[20,21] There is also a possible association with connective tissue diseases such as Ehlers-Danlos syndrome, Marfan syndrome, and Loeys-Dietz syndrome.[22] This finding suggests that the suspicion for EoE should be heightened in individuals with such diseases.

PATHOPHYSIOLOGY

EoE shares many immunologic features with other atopic diseases. In addition to local eosinophilia, studies from human and animal models have shown that EoE is characterized by impaired epithelial barrier function[23,24] and infiltration of T helper type 2 (Th2) $CD4^+$ helper T cells,[25,26] mast cells,[27] basophils,[28] plasma cells,[29] and group 2 innate lymphoid cells.[30] Although allergen-specific IgE antibodies are also often detected, elimination diets based solely on IgE sensitization have had mixed success,[31,32] and the use of anti-IgE treatment was not shown to be more efficacious in inducing EoE remission than placebo.[29] It has been shown, in both pediatric and adult populations, however, that food is a key trigger for EoE.[33,34] The strongest such evidence comes from trials with elemental diets, where histologic remission rates of greater than 90% are observed, although focused food elimination diets also often lead to remission.[10,11,34] Taken together, EoE is often considered a non–IgE-mediated, food antigen–driven hypersensitivity,[35] although the exact mechanism remains unclear.

Candidate and unbiased genetic approaches have identified a number of genes associated with EoE. These include the genes that encode for (or are involved in the regulation of) thymic stromal lymphopoietin, filaggrin, desmoglein-1, calpain-14, eotaxin-3, and transforming growth factor-β.[36] Many of these genes are known to be involved in the regulation of barrier function, Th2 induction, and tissue remodeling. Consistent with a Th2-related inflammatory milieu, the cytokines interleukin (IL)-4, IL-5, and IL-13 are also upregulated in EoE.[37] Emerging data also show abundant antigen-specific immunoglobulin G4 (IgG4) in the esophageal mucosa and peripheral blood.[29,38] To date, the relative importance of these different cellular and molecular mediators in the pathogenesis of EoE remains to be established.

DIAGNOSTIC TESTS

EoE is a clinicopathologic disease and, thus, the diagnosis depends on certain pathologic findings in individuals with an appropriate clinical history. As such, an esophagogastroduodenoscopy is a required part of the workup for EoE. At the macroscopic level, a number of findings are associated with EoE, including esophageal rings, linear furrows, plaques, stenosis, and strictures; however, these findings are neither sensitive nor specific for this disease.[39] Histologic evidence of at least 15 eosinophils per high-power field on esophageal mucosal biopsy is required for diagnosis. Based on current guidelines, the diagnosis requires that the elevated eosinophils be limited to the esophagus and not be due to other underlying causes of eosinophilia. Furthermore, this esophageal eosinophilia must be present despite 8 weeks of empiric therapy with a protein pump inhibitor (PPI).[40] In those for whom there is a favorable response to a PPI (ie, the eosinophils decrease to <15 per high-power field on repeat endoscopy), the label PPI-responsive esophageal eosinophilia (PPI-REE) is applied. Previous studies, however, demonstrate similar clinical,[41] histologic, immunologic,[42,43] and molecular[44] characteristics between patients with PPI-REE and EoE, and thus there are currently conflicting opinions as to whether PPI-REE signifies a truly unique pathophysiologic state, or whether it should be considered within the spectrum of EoE.[45,46] As such, recently published European guidelines have eliminated the criteria for a PPI challenge before diagnosing EoE.[1]

The role for allergy evaluation is important for both the management of EoE and that of comorbid atopic conditions, such as asthma, allergic rhinitis, IgE-mediated food allergy, and atopic dermatitis, which affect a majority of individuals with EoE.[47–49] Individuals with EoE frequently experience allergic rhinitis symptoms and may have seasonal exacerbations of their EoE,[50–52] and thus a thorough evaluation of aeroallergen sensitization and treatment of allergic rhinitis symptoms is recommended. Furthermore, children with EoE frequently have concomitant IgE-mediated food allergy,[19] and thus a careful evaluation of this condition, especially in light of possible elimination diets and food reintroduction, is essential.

As mentioned, previous studies examining the use of elemental diets in both children and adults with EoE have demonstrated histologic remission in more than 90% of patients,[10,11] suggesting that exposure to certain foods are a key trigger for this condition. However, because elemental diets are burdensome and unappealing to many individuals, efforts have focused on the utility of allergy testing, such as skin prick tests, patch tests, and quantification of food-specific IgE, to design more tailored avoidance diets. In general, studies examining allergy testing–directed diets have shown mixed results, albeit with outcomes inferior to elemental diets (**Table 1**). A recent metaanalysis demonstrated that 45% of individuals responded to diets guided by allergy testing, but there was considerable heterogeneity among the studies, which likely reflects different testing approaches.[34]

The majority of studies examining allergy testing–directed diets have assessed the utility of using positive results from both skin prick and atopy patch testing. Atopy patch testing involves the topical application of fresh food to the skin for 48 hours, with subsequent evaluation and follow-up at 72 hours. Atopy patch testing is an intuitive approach given that IgE-independent mechanisms are thought to be involved in EoE, but the testing is logistically challenging and has not been shown to be universally successful.[53–55]

The predictive value of testing serum for food-specific IgE is less well-studied than skin testing, but recent reports suggest that low-level, specific IgE may be useful for dietary guidance.[56,57] The fact that testing for specific IgE by a multiarray component assay was not helpful likely reflects important differences between traditional ImmunoCAP assays and multiarray component assays,[14] with ImmunoCAP having greater sensitivity to many food allergens.[58] It has been theorized that this poor correlation may be due to assay inhibition by IgG4-blocking antibodies.[59,60] A role for food-specific IgG4 in identifying food triggers remains an open question; a recent study also demonstrated that food-specific IgG4 levels of trigger foods decrease significantly in patients with EoE after dietary elimination of these foods.[38] However, whether this test may be used to predict causative foods remains unclear.

Table 1
Key studies assessing the utility of allergy testing in eosinophilic esophagitis

Study (Year)	Testing Modality	No. of Subjects	Histologic Response (%)	Additional Findings
Children				
Spergel et al,[31] 2002	SPT and APT	26	75[a]	Prospective study Milk and egg were the most common positive foods by SPT Wheat was the most common positive food by APT
Spergel et al,[53] 2005	SPT and APT	146	49[b]	Retrospective analysis of clinic population Egg, milk, and soy were most common trigger foods identified by SPT Corn, soy, and wheat were most common foods identified by APT
Spergel et al,[32] 2012	SPT and APT	319	53[b]	Retrospective analysis of clinic population Of 941 patients, causative foods were identified in 319 Similar histologic success for SPT/APT directed diets and SFED Most common trigger foods were milk, egg, wheat, and soy
Al-Hussaini et al,[102] 2013	SPT and food-specific IgE (ImmunoCAP > 0.35 kU/L)	10	40[c]	Prospective study Most common trigger foods were milk, soy, wheat, egg, and nuts
Henderson et al,[54] 2012	SPT and APT	23	65[c]	Retrospective comparison of elemental, SFED, and allergy testing directed diets Elemental diet was the most effective SFED and allergy testing directed diets had comparable effectiveness
Adults				
Molina-Infante et al,[55] 2012	SPT, APT, and prick-prick testing	15	33[d]	Prospective trial Foods that were positive by any form of testing were eliminated
Wolf et al,[103] 2014	SPT	22	32[a]	Retrospective study of clinic cohort Milk, egg, and wheat were most common trigger foods

(continued on next page)

Table 1
(continued)

Study (Year)	Testing Modality	No. of Subjects	Histologic Response (%)	Additional Findings
Rodriguez-Sanchez et al,[56] 2014	Food-specific IgE (ImmunoCAP >0.1 kU/L)	26	73[d]	Compared SFED to sIgE-targeted diets. Fewer foods were removed and fewer EGDs were required in sIgE-directed diet Most common triggers: milk, wheat, egg, and legumes
Van Rhijn et al,[104] 2015	Component IgE (ImmunoCAP ISAC)	15	7[e]	Prospective trial of IgE-directed diet, based on ISAC assay Trial was prematurely terminated because only 1 of 15 patients showed improvement in the interim analysis

Abbreviations: APT, atopy patch testing; EGD, esophagogastroduodenoscopy; IgE, immunoglobulin E; ISAC, immuno-solid phase allergen chip; SFED, 6-food elimination diet; sIgE, allergen-specific immunoglobulin E; SPT, skin prick testing.
[a] Based on resolution of symptoms and biopsy results when available.
[b] Less than 5 eosinophils per high-power field.
[c] Less than 15 eosinophils per high-power field.
[d] Less than 14 eosinophils per high-power field and clinical improvement.
[e] Less than 10 eosinophils per high-power field.

DIFFERENTIAL DIAGNOSIS

The differential diagnosis for EoE includes a number of conditions that can cause esophageal eosinophilia and upper gastrointestinal symptoms. These include gastroesophageal reflux, parasitic or fungal infections, connective tissue disease, Crohn's disease, celiac disease, carcinoma, drug-related eosinophilia, congenital rings, achalasia, vasculitis and bullous pemphigoid. It is important to exclude these entities based on history and, in some cases, complementary testing.

TREATMENT

Evidence-based treatment options for EoE generally fall into one of the following categories: Acid suppression, dietary avoidance, swallowed steroids, or esophageal dilation. With current guidelines requiring PPI failure as part of EoE diagnostic criteria, an obvious implication is that acid suppression by itself is inadequate therapy (with the exception of PPI-REE). However, as discussed, recent European guidelines have eliminated the requirement of a PPI trial before the diagnosis of EoE, and thus treatment with a PPI alone may be adequate in select patients.[1] The decision of whether to continue a PPI after confirming the diagnosis of EoE is not clear cut, but may be considered if the PPI nonetheless improves symptoms such as reflux or dysphagia.[61] The decision to continue a PPI should be made after weighing the benefits versus the risks associated with the long-term use of these medications.[62,63]

Most patients initially start therapy with either dietary avoidance or a topical steroid. Oral steroids or immunosuppressants can be considered for severe cases, but these agents are not commonly used or recommended.[64] The advantage of dietary avoidance is that it avoids complications that can result from long-term topical steroid use, such as esophageal candidiasis,[65,66] cataracts,[67] and adrenal suppression.[68] A disadvantage is that long-term diet restrictions can be challenging, particularly if there are multiple trigger foods. There have been few head-to-head trials comparing food elimination and steroids, although a recent report by Philpott and colleagues[69] agrees with our clinical experience that steroids may be more likely to achieve remission than diet alone. Often we find that patients have strong preferences for one option or the other, which helps to guide initial management.

Approaches to dietary avoidance can be empiric elimination of the most common food triggers, allergy testing–directed diets, or elemental diets. The fact that allergy tests have not consistently proven useful for predicting trigger foods has led many providers to start with empiric diets. The classic 6-food elimination diet (SFED) involves avoidance of milk, wheat, egg, soy, fish/shellfish, and peanuts/tree nuts. This diet was initially studied, in large part, because these foods are commonly associated with IgE-mediated food allergy[70]; however, numerous studies have shown that the SFED can be effective in EoE as well (**Table 2**).[71] Studies examining the SFED have generally shown histologic remission in 60% to 80% of cases,[54,70,72] which is also supported by findings in the systematic review and metaanalysis by Arias and colleagues.[34]

Two recent studies have evaluated the efficacy of an empiric 4-food elimination diet. In the first study, which was performed in adults, avoidance of milk/dairy, gluten-containing grains, egg, and legumes led to remission in 54% of patients.[73] It is important to note that this "4-food elimination diet" also included avoidance of goat and sheep's milk, all gluten-containing grains, lentils, chickpeas, peas, beans, peanuts, and many tree nuts. More recently, avoidance of milk, dairy products, wheat, egg, and soy was assessed in children with EoE, and a similar percentage of patients (65%) achieved histologic remission.[74]

With the realization that milk and wheat are the most common triggers, some investigators have transitioned to a 'step-up' approach, which involves starting with avoidance of milk and gluten-containing cereals, and only restricting additional foods if there has been a response failure.[75] It is important to note, however, that foods that are not included in the SFED have also been implicated in some studies.[19,31,76]

The topical steroid formulations that have been most studied are budesonide and fluticasone. Although neither agent is approved by the US Food and Drug Administration for the treatment of EoE, both have shown efficacy in controlled trials, and treatment with these medications is supported by American College of Gastroenterology guidelines.[40] Fluticasone is usually administered twice a day with a metered-dose inhaler without a spacer. Although the optimal dose has not been established, commonly used doses are 176 µg/d in 1 to 4-year-old children, 440 µg/d in children 5- to 10-year-old children, and 880 to 1760 µg/d for those 11 years or older,[77] although some investigators have used 1760 µg/d in children as young as 3 years of age.[78] It is critical that the patient swallow and not inhale the medication. Some providers advocate ingesting the contents of individually wrapped foil-lined packets within the dry powder inhaler formulation of fluticasone for easier delivery.[79] Budesonide can be administered by ingestion of the nebulized formulation, but most providers favor using a viscous slurry. In this case, the content of a budesonide respule is added to a thickening agent, such as sucralose, although other vehicles including honey, agave nectar, Neocate Nutra, and applesauce are also frequently used.[80,81] Typically,

Table 2
Key studies assessing utility of empiric diets in eosinophilic esophagitis

Study (Year)	Empiric Diet	No. of Subjects	Histologic Response (%)	Additional Findings
Children				
Kagalwalla et al,[70] 2006	SFED	35	74[a]	Retrospective observational study comparing SFED with elemental formula diet Established that the SFED is associated with clinical and histologic improvement in eosinophilic esophagitis
Henderson et al,[54] 2012		26	81[b]	Retrospective comparison of elemental, SFED, and allergy-testing directed diets, as outlined in **Table 1**
Kagalwalla et al,[74] 2017	FFED	78	64	Prospective observational study Patients with detectable specific IgE (>0.35 IU/mL) were less likely to respond to diet
Kagalwalla et al,[105] 2012	Milk only	17	65[b]	Retrospective study of clinic cohort
Erwin et al,[57] 2016		21	62[b]	Prospective observational study Demonstrated that patients with low, and even undetectable, specific IgE to milk responded to milk elimination diet
Adults				
Gonsalves et al,[72] 2012	SFED	50	74[b]	First study of SFED in adults Most common triggers were wheat and milk SPT only predicted trigger foods in 13%
Lucendo et al,[76] 2013		67	73[b]	Also excluded rice, corn, and legumes 15 patients demonstrated remission at 2 years Most common triggers were milk, wheat, eggs, and legumes
Rodriguez-Sanchez et al,[56] 2014		17	53[b]	Compared SFED with sIgE-targeted diets, as outlined in **Table 1**
Philpott et al,[69] 2016		56	52[b]	Prospective, observational study in Australia comparing SFED with swallowed budesonide
Molina-Infante et al,[73] 2014	FFED	52	54[b]	SFED successful in 31% of FFED nonresponders Milk was the most common trigger (50%)

Abbreviations: FFED, 4-food elimination diet; IgE, immunoglobulin E; SFED, 6-food elimination diet; sIgE, allergen-specific immunoglobulin E.
[a] Less than 10 eosinophils per high-power field.
[b] Less than 15 eosinophils per high-power field.

1 mg of budesonide will be mixed with 0.5 to 1.0 teaspoons of sweetener.[81] The recommended oral viscous budesonide dose in children (<10 years old) is 1 mg once a day, and in those older than 10 years, it is 1 mg twice a day. For both fluticasone and budesonide, it is recommended that food and drink be avoided for at least 30 minutes after administration. There have been no head-to-head trials comparing the 2 different steroid preparations, but an intriguing trial compared budesonide by the viscous versus nebulized formulations and found that viscous budesonide was superior for reducing eosinophilic inflammation.[82] Not unexpectedly, scintigraphy analysis demonstrated that the viscous formulation had extended contact with the esophageal mucosa compared with the nebulized version. Moreover, a recent retrospective comparison of the experience at a single center showed EoE subjects treated with oral viscous budesonide achieved histologic remission (75%) more often than those treated with swallowed fluticasone (40%).[83] Taken together, these studies suggest that budesonide viscous slurry may be of benefit in individuals who have failed fluticasone.

A final option to be considered in some cases is periodic esophageal dilation. Some individuals with esophageal strictures may require dilation as part of a multifaceted treatment approach. In other cases, primarily when symptoms are restricted to dysphagia owing to strictures, the symptoms may be addressed solely through periodic esophageal dilation. This approach is undertaken with the important caveat that the procedure is not addressing the underlying inflammation. Dilation has been shown to be successful in many studies, with a recent metaanalysis showing improvement in 75% of cases.[84] The possibility of adverse events, including postprocedural chest pain, esophageal perforation, and hemorrhage, must be considered when dilation is considered.[84]

MANAGEMENT

The natural history of EoE is not completely understood, but it is thought to be a chronic disease, and the development of fibrotic changes and strictures seems to be common in those with delayed diagnosis.[85] Because symptoms and histologic inflammation have been shown to recur in individuals who stop treatment, continued management and surveillance of patients is recommended.[40] In particular, maintenance therapy with swallowed steroids or dietary management should be considered in patients with severe dysphagia, a history of food impaction, high-grade esophageal strictures, and a rapid clinical or histologic response with therapy.[40]

Although long-term outcomes are not well-established, there is evidence that dietary elimination can lead to sustained remission in those who successfully avoid their food triggers.[76] In these patients, especially those avoiding multiple foods, it is important to monitor for nutritional deficiencies and to strongly consider referral to or comanagement with a dietitian.

Maintenance therapy with swallowed steroids was evaluated in a prospective study of 28 adults with EoE in remission who were treated with either twice daily budesonide (0.25 mg) or placebo for 50 weeks. Although eosinophil counts increased in both groups during the study, the increase was statistically less among those treated with swallowed budesonide compared with those treated with placebo, and it was not associated with a significant increase in clinical symptoms.[86] In the absence of long-term data, the risks of treating with swallowed steroids remain largely theoretical, but emerging data suggest a need for careful monitoring of adverse effects. For example, in a prospective trial of children with EoE who were treated with topical steroids for a mean duration of 15 weeks, 66% of children developed adrenal suppression.[87] For this reason, periodic monitoring of a morning cortisol level or adrenocorticotrophic hormone is suggested. To minimize the long-term risk of steroids, the dose should ideally be reduced to the minimum that will achieve ongoing remission of symptoms and inflammation; however, this strategy is complicated by emerging evidence that dose reduction often leads to a loss of response.[78,88]

FUTURE CONSIDERATIONS

Two key areas of ongoing investigation in EoE relate to the development of novel diagnostics and therapeutics. The current reliance on esophagogastroduodenoscopy for diagnosis and management of EoE has several pitfalls. An important one is that the inflammatory lesions in EoE are often patchy, which means that several samples are required to reduce the chance of a false negative. And although generally very safe, EGDs are invasive and expensive procedures that carry the risk of infection, perforation, and adverse effects from anesthesia. Novel approaches that may impact diagnosis and/or surveillance include a microarray gene expression diagnostic panel[89] and noninvasive techniques that use a capsule or sponge to measure luminal secretions.[90,91] Given the limitations of our current allergy testing, the development of novel assays to identify food and environmental triggers of EoE would further have an important role in guiding more personalized avoidance strategies.

From a therapeutic perspective, there is ongoing interest in targeting a number of mediators involved in eosinophil recruitment and Th2 inflammation. One of the most studied targets to date is IL-5, a cytokine important in the maturation and recruitment of eosinophils.[92] Mepolizumab[93–95] and reslizumab,[96] both monoclonal antibodies targeting IL-5, have been shown in clinical trials to decrease esophageal eosinophilia, but clinical responses have not been uniform. Similarly, a monoclonal antibody targeting IL-13, a Th2 cytokine that is increased in the esophagi of patients with EoE,[97] was found to significantly decrease esophageal eosinophils, and there was a nonsignificant trend toward improved symptoms.[98] A clinical trial of an inhibitor of chemoattractant receptor-homologous molecule on Th2 cells, which is expressed by pathogenic effector Th2 cells,[99] was also shown to reduce esophageal eosinophilia and improve clinical symptoms.[100] Potential future targets that may prove efficacious in treating EoE include monoclonal antibodies against IL-4 receptor alpha, a shared receptor for both IL-4 and IL-13, thymic stromal lymphopoietin, and IL-9.[101]

SUMMARY

EoE is an emerging chronic inflammatory disease with significant associated morbidity. EoE is commonly food triggered, and appropriate dietary avoidance is often sufficient for disease remission. Ongoing research holds great promise for the development of novel tools for disease diagnosis and management, as well as for the development of targeted therapies.

REFERENCES

1. Lucendo AJ, Molina-Infante J, Arias A, et al. Guidelines on eosinophilic esophagitis: evidence-based statements and recommendations for diagnosis and management in children and adults. United European Gastroenterol J 2017; 5(3):335–58.

2. Attwood SE, Smyrk TC, Demeester TR, et al. Esophageal eosinophilia with dysphagia. A distinct clinicopathologic syndrome. Dig Dis Sci 1993;38(1): 109–16.

3. Straumann A, Spichtin HP, Bernoulli R, et al. Idiopathic eosinophilic esophagitis: a frequently overlooked disease with typical clinical aspects and discrete endoscopic findings. Schweiz Med Wochenschr 1994;124(33):1419–29 [in German].

4. Dellon ES. Epidemiology of eosinophilic esophagitis. Gastroenterol Clin North Am 2014;43(2):201–18.

5. Hruz P, Straumann A, Bussmann C, et al. Escalating incidence of eosinophilic esophagitis: a 20-year prospective, population-based study in Olten County, Switzerland. J Allergy Clin Immunol 2011;128(6):1349–50.e5.

6. Prasad GA, Alexander JA, Schleck CD, et al. Epidemiology of eosinophilic esophagitis over three decades in Olmsted County, Minnesota. Clin Gastroenterol Hepatol 2009;7(10):1055–61.

7. Jensen ET, Martin CF, Kappelman MD, et al. Prevalence of eosinophilic gastritis, gastroenteritis, and colitis: estimates from a national administrative database. J Pediatr Gastroenterol Nutr 2016;62(1):36–42.

8. Dellon ES, Erichsen R, Baron JA, et al. The increasing incidence and prevalence of eosinophilic oesophagitis outpaces changes in endoscopic and biopsy practice: national population-based estimates from Denmark. Aliment Pharmacol Ther 2015;41(7):662–70.

9. Giriens B, Yan P, Safroneeva E, et al. Escalating incidence of eosinophilic esophagitis in Canton of Vaud, Switzerland, 1993-2013: a population-based study. Allergy 2015;70(12):1633–9.

10. Kelly KJ, Lazenby AJ, Rowe PC, et al. Eosinophilic esophagitis attributed to gastroesophageal reflux: improvement with an amino acid-based formula. Gastroenterology 1995;109(5):1503–12.

11. Peterson KA, Byrne KR, Vinson LA, et al. Elemental diet induces histologic response in adult eosinophilic esophagitis. Am J Gastroenterol 2013;108(5): 759–66.

12. Sorser SA, Barawi M, Hagglund K, et al. Eosinophilic esophagitis in children and adolescents: epidemiology, clinical presentation and seasonal variation. J Gastroenterol 2013;48(1):81–5.

13. Spergel JM, Brown-Whitehorn TF, Beausoleil JL, et al. 14 years of eosinophilic esophagitis: clinical features and prognosis. J Pediatr Gastroenterol Nutr 2009;48(1):30–6.

14. Erwin EA, Tripathi A, Ogbogu PU, et al. IgE antibody detection and component analysis in patients with eosinophilic esophagitis. J Allergy Clin Immunol Pract 2015;3(6):896–904.e3.

15. Miehlke S. Clinical features of Eosinophilic esophagitis in children and adults. Best Pract Res Clin Gastroenterol 2015;29(5):739–48.

16. Lucendo AJ, Castillo P, Martin-Chavarri S, et al. Manometric findings in adult eosinophilic oesophagitis: a study of 12 cases. Eur J Gastroenterol Hepatol 2007;19(5):417–24.

17. Garcia-Compean D, Gonzalez Gonzalez JA, Marrufo Garcia CA, et al. Prevalence of eosinophilic esophagitis in patients with refractory gastroesophageal reflux disease symptoms: a prospective study. Dig Liver Dis 2011;43(3):204–8.

18. Simon D, Marti H, Heer P, et al. Eosinophilic esophagitis is frequently associated with IgE-mediated allergic airway diseases. J Allergy Clin Immunol 2005;115(5): 1090–2.

19. Hill DA, Dudley JW, Spergel JM. The prevalence of eosinophilic esophagitis in pediatric patients with IgE-mediated food allergy. J Allergy Clin Immunol Pract 2017;5(2):369–75.

20. Padia R, Curtin K, Peterson K, et al. Eosinophilic esophagitis strongly linked to chronic rhinosinusitis. Laryngoscope 2016;126(6):1279–83.

21. Peterson K, Firszt R, Fang J, et al. Risk of autoimmunity in EoE and families: a population-based cohort study. Am J Gastroenterol 2016;111(7):926–32.

22. Abonia JP, Wen T, Stucke EM, et al. High prevalence of eosinophilic esophagitis in patients with inherited connective tissue disorders. J Allergy Clin Immunol 2013;132(2):378–86.

23. Davis BP, Stucke EM, Khorki ME, et al. Eosinophilic esophagitis-linked calpain 14 is an IL-13-induced protease that mediates esophageal epithelial barrier impairment. JCI Insight 2016;1(4):e86355.

24. Simon D, Radonjic-Hosli S, Straumann A, et al. Active eosinophilic esophagitis is characterized by epithelial barrier defects and eosinophil extracellular trap formation. Allergy 2015;70(4):443–52.

25. Straumann A, Bauer M, Fischer B, et al. Idiopathic eosinophilic esophagitis is associated with a T(H)2-type allergic inflammatory response. J Allergy Clin Immunol 2001;108(6):954–61.

26. Yamazaki K, Murray JA, Arora AS, et al. Allergen-specific in vitro cytokine production in adult patients with eosinophilic esophagitis. Dig Dis Sci 2006; 51(11):1934–41.

27. Arias A, Lucendo AJ, Martinez-Fernandez P, et al. Dietary treatment modulates mast cell phenotype, density, and activity in adult eosinophilic oesophagitis. Clin Exp Allergy 2016;46(1):78–91.

28. Noti M, Wojno ED, Kim BS, et al. Thymic stromal lymphopoietin-elicited basophil responses promote eosinophilic esophagitis. Nat Med 2013;19(8):1005–13.

29. Clayton F, Fang JC, Gleich GJ, et al. Eosinophilic esophagitis in adults is associated with IgG4 and not mediated by IgE. Gastroenterology 2014;147(3): 602–9.

30. Doherty TA, Baum R, Newbury RO, et al. Group 2 innate lymphocytes (ILC2) are enriched in active eosinophilic esophagitis. J Allergy Clin Immunol 2015;136(3): 792–4.e3.

31. Spergel JM, Beausoleil JL, Mascarenhas M, et al. The use of skin prick tests and patch tests to identify causative foods in eosinophilic esophagitis. J Allergy Clin Immunol 2002;109(2):363–8.

32. Spergel JM, Brown-Whitehorn TF, Cianferoni A, et al. Identification of causative foods in children with eosinophilic esophagitis treated with an elimination diet. J Allergy Clin Immunol 2012;130(2):461–7.e5.

33. McGowan EC, Platts-Mills TA. Eosinophilic esophagitis from an allergy perspective: how to optimally pursue allergy testing & dietary modification in the adult population. Curr Gastroenterol Rep 2016;18(11):58.

34. Arias A, Gonzalez-Cervera J, Tenias JM, et al. Efficacy of dietary interventions for inducing histologic remission in patients with eosinophilic esophagitis: a systematic review and meta-analysis. Gastroenterology 2014;146(7):1639–48.

35. Simon D, Cianferoni A, Spergel JM, et al. Eosinophilic esophagitis is characterized by a non-IgE-mediated food hypersensitivity. Allergy 2016;71(5):611–20.

36. Davis BP, Rothenberg ME. Mechanisms of disease of eosinophilic esophagitis. Annu Rev Pathol 2016;11:365–93.

37. Blanchard C, Stucke EM, Rodriguez-Jimenez B, et al. A striking local esophageal cytokine expression profile in eosinophilic esophagitis. J Allergy Clin Immunol 2011;127(1):208–17, 217.e-7.
38. Wright BL, Kulis M, Guo R, et al. Food-specific IgG4 is associated with eosinophilic esophagitis. J Allergy Clin Immunol 2016;138(4):1190–2.e3.
39. Miehlke S. Clinical features of eosinophilic esophagitis. Dig Dis 2014;32(1–2): 61–7.
40. Dellon ES, Gonsalves N, Hirano I, et al. ACG clinical guideline: evidenced based approach to the diagnosis and management of esophageal eosinophilia and eosinophilic esophagitis (EoE). Am J Gastroenterol 2013;108(5):679–92 [quiz: 693].
41. Molina-Infante J, Ferrando-Lamana L, Ripoll C, et al. Esophageal eosinophilic infiltration responds to proton pump inhibition in most adults. Clin Gastroenterol Hepatol 2011;9(2):110–7.
42. Moawad FJ, Wells JM, Johnson RL, et al. Comparison of eotaxin-3 biomarker in patients with eosinophilic oesophagitis, proton pump inhibitor-responsive oesophageal eosinophilia and gastro-oesophageal reflux disease. Aliment Pharmacol Ther 2015;42(2):231–8.
43. Molina-Infante J, Rivas MD, Hernandez-Alonso M, et al. Proton pump inhibitor-responsive oesophageal eosinophilia correlates with downregulation of eotaxin-3 and Th2 cytokines overexpression. Aliment Pharmacol Ther 2014; 40(8):955–65.
44. Wen T, Dellon ES, Moawad FJ, et al. Transcriptome analysis of proton pump inhibitor-responsive esophageal eosinophilia reveals proton pump inhibitor-reversible allergic inflammation. J Allergy Clin Immunol 2015;135(1):187–97.
45. Shoda T, Matsuda A, Nomura I, et al. Eosinophilic esophagitis vs proton pump inhibitor-responsive esophageal eosinophilia: transcriptome analysis. J Allergy Clin Immunol 2010;139(6):2010–3.
46. Molina-Infante J, Bredenoord AJ, Cheng E, et al. Proton pump inhibitor-responsive oesophageal eosinophilia: an entity challenging current diagnostic criteria for eosinophilic oesophagitis. Gut 2016;65(3):524–31.
47. Orenstein SR, Shalaby TM, Di Lorenzo C, et al. The spectrum of pediatric eosinophilic esophagitis beyond infancy: a clinical series of 30 children. Am J Gastroenterol 2000;95(6):1422–30.
48. Roy-Ghanta S, Larosa DF, Katzka DA. Atopic characteristics of adult patients with eosinophilic esophagitis. Clin Gastroenterol Hepatol 2008;6(5):531–5.
49. Gonzalez-Cervera J, Arias A, Redondo-Gonzalez O, et al. Association between atopic manifestations and eosinophilic esophagitis: a systematic review and meta-analysis. Ann Allergy Asthma Immunol 2017;118(5):582–90.e2.
50. Almansa C, Krishna M, Buchner AM, et al. Seasonal distribution in newly diagnosed cases of eosinophilic esophagitis in adults. Am J Gastroenterol 2009; 104(4):828–33.
51. Moawad FJ, Veerappan GR, Lake JM, et al. Correlation between eosinophilic oesophagitis and aeroallergens. Aliment Pharmacol Ther 2010;31(4):509–15.
52. Fahey L, Robinson G, Weinberger K, et al. Correlation between aeroallergen levels and new diagnosis of eosinophilic esophagitis in New York city. J Pediatr Gastroenterol Nutr 2017;64(1):22–5.
53. Spergel JM, Andrews T, Brown-Whitehorn TF, et al. Treatment of eosinophilic esophagitis with specific food elimination diet directed by a combination of skin prick and patch tests. Ann Allergy Asthma Immunol 2005;95(4):336–43.

54. Henderson CJ, Abonia JP, King EC, et al. Comparative dietary therapy effectiveness in remission of pediatric eosinophilic esophagitis. J Allergy Clin Immunol 2012;129(6):1570–8.

55. Molina-Infante J, Martin-Noguerol E, Alvarado-Arenas M, et al. Selective elimination diet based on skin testing has suboptimal efficacy for adult eosinophilic esophagitis. J Allergy Clin Immunol 2012;130(5):1200–2.

56. Rodriguez-Sanchez J, Gomez Torrijos E, Lopez Viedma B, et al. Efficacy of IgE-targeted vs empiric six-food elimination diets for adult eosinophilic oesophagitis. Allergy 2014;69(7):936–42.

57. Erwin EA, Kruszewski PG, Russo JM, et al. IgE antibodies and response to cow's milk elimination diet in pediatric eosinophilic esophagitis. J Allergy Clin Immunol 2016;138(2):625–8.e2.

58. Sastre J. Molecular diagnosis in allergy. Clin Exp Allergy 2010;40(10):1442–60.

59. Aalberse RC, Platts-Mills TA, Rispens T. The developmental history of IgE and IgG4 antibodies in relation to atopy, eosinophilic esophagitis, and the modified TH2 response. Curr Allergy Asthma Rep 2016;16(6):45.

60. Dellon ES. Diagnostics of eosinophilic esophagitis: clinical, endoscopic, and histologic pitfalls. Dig Dis 2014;32(1–2):48–53.

61. Asher Wolf W, Dellon ES. Eosinophilic esophagitis and proton pump inhibitors: controversies and implications for clinical practice. Gastroenterol Hepatol (N Y) 2014;10(7):427–32.

62. Schnoll-Sussman F, Katz PO. Clinical implications of emerging data on the safety of proton pump inhibitors. Curr Treat Options Gastroenterol 2017;15(1): 1–9.

63. Scarpignato C, Gatta L, Zullo A, et al. Effective and safe proton pump inhibitor therapy in acid-related diseases - a position paper addressing benefits and potential harms of acid suppression. BMC Med 2016;14(1):179.

64. Netzer P, Gschossmann JM, Straumann A, et al. Corticosteroid-dependent eosinophilic oesophagitis: azathioprine and 6-mercaptopurine can induce and maintain long-term remission. Eur J Gastroenterol Hepatol 2007;19(10):865–9.

65. Chuang MY, Chinnaratha MA, Hancock DG, et al. Topical steroid therapy for the treatment of eosinophilic esophagitis (EoE): a systematic review and meta-analysis. Clin Transl Gastroenterol 2015;6:e82.

66. Miehlke S, Hruz P, Vieth M, et al. A randomised, double-blind trial comparing budesonide formulations and dosages for short-term treatment of eosinophilic oesophagitis. Gut 2016;65(3):390–9.

67. Weatherall M, Clay J, James K, et al. Dose-response relationship of inhaled corticosteroids and cataracts: a systematic review and meta-analysis. Respirology 2009;14(7):983–90.

68. Harel S, Hursh BE, Chan ES, et al. Adrenal suppression in children treated with oral viscous budesonide for eosinophilic esophagitis. J Pediatr Gastroenterol Nutr 2015;61(2):190–3.

69. Philpott H, Nandurkar S, Royce SG, et al. Allergy tests do not predict food triggers in adult patients with eosinophilic oesophagitis. A comprehensive prospective study using five modalities. Aliment Pharmacol Ther 2016;44(3):223–33.

70. Kagalwalla AF, Sentongo TA, Ritz S, et al. Effect of six-food elimination diet on clinical and histologic outcomes in eosinophilic esophagitis. Clin Gastroenterol Hepatol 2006;4(9):1097–102.

71. Boyce JA, Assa'ad A, Burks AW, et al. Guidelines for the diagnosis and management of food allergy in the United States: summary of the NIAID-sponsored expert panel report. J Allergy Clin Immunol 2010;126(6):1105–18.

72. Gonsalves N, Yang GY, Doerfler B, et al. Elimination diet effectively treats eosinophilic esophagitis in adults; food reintroduction identifies causative factors. Gastroenterology 2012;142(7):1451–9.e1 [quiz: e14–5].
73. Molina-Infante J, Arias A, Barrio J, et al. Four-food group elimination diet for adult eosinophilic esophagitis: a prospective multicenter study. J Allergy Clin Immunol 2014;134(5):1093–9.e1.
74. Kagalwalla AF, Wechsler JB, Amsden K, et al. Efficacy of a 4-food elimination diet for children with eosinophilic esophagitis. Clin Gastroenterol Hepatol 2017. [Epub ahead of print].
75. Molina-Infante J, Gonzalez-Cordero PL, Arias A, et al. Update on dietary therapy for eosinophilic esophagitis in children and adults. Expert Rev Gastroenterol Hepatol 2017;11(2):115–23.
76. Lucendo AJ, Arias A, Gonzalez-Cervera J, et al. Empiric 6-food elimination diet induced and maintained prolonged remission in patients with adult eosinophilic esophagitis: a prospective study on the food cause of the disease. J Allergy Clin Immunol 2013;131(3):797–804.
77. Teitelbaum JE, Fox VL, Twarog FJ, et al. Eosinophilic esophagitis in children: immunopathological analysis and response to fluticasone propionate. Gastroenterology 2002;122(5):1216–25.
78. Butz BK, Wen T, Gleich GJ, et al. Efficacy, dose reduction, and resistance to high-dose fluticasone in patients with eosinophilic esophagitis. Gastroenterology 2014;147(2):324–33.e5.
79. Hirano I. How I approach the management of eosinophilic esophagitis in adults. Am J Gastroenterol 2017;112(2):197–9.
80. Lee J, Shuker M, Brown-Whitehorn T, et al. Oral viscous budesonide can be successfully delivered through a variety of vehicles to treat eosinophilic esophagitis in children. J Allergy Clin Immunol Pract 2016;4(4):767–8.
81. Rubinstein E, Lee JJ, Fried A, et al. Comparison of 2 delivery vehicles for viscous budesonide to treat eosinophilic esophagitis in children. J Pediatr Gastroenterol Nutr 2014;59(3):317–20.
82. Dellon ES, Sheikh A, Speck O, et al. Viscous topical is more effective than nebulized steroid therapy for patients with eosinophilic esophagitis. Gastroenterology 2012;143(2):321–4.e1.
83. Fable JM, Fernandez M, Goodine S, et al. Retrospective comparison of fluticasone propionate and oral viscous budesonide in children with eosinophilic esophagitis. J Pediatr Gastroenterol Nutr 2017. [Epub ahead of print].
84. Moawad FJ, Cheatham JG, DeZee KJ. Meta-analysis: the safety and efficacy of dilation in eosinophilic oesophagitis. Aliment Pharmacol Ther 2013;38(7):713–20.
85. Schoepfer AM, Safroneeva E, Bussmann C, et al. Delay in diagnosis of eosinophilic esophagitis increases risk for stricture formation in a time-dependent manner. Gastroenterology 2013;145(6):1230–6.e1-2.
86. Straumann A, Conus S, Degen L, et al. Long-term budesonide maintenance treatment is partially effective for patients with eosinophilic esophagitis. Clin Gastroenterol Hepatol 2011;9(5):400–9.e1.
87. Ahmet A, Benchimol EI, Goldbloom EB, et al. Adrenal suppression in children treated with swallowed fluticasone and oral viscous budesonide for eosinophilic esophagitis. Allergy Asthma Clin Immunol 2016;12:49.
88. Eluri S, Runge TM, Hansen J, et al. Diminishing effectiveness of long-term maintenance topical steroid therapy in PPI non-responsive eosinophilic esophagitis. Clin Transl Gastroenterol 2017;8(6):e97.

89. Wen T, Stucke EM, Grotjan TM, et al. Molecular diagnosis of eosinophilic esophagitis by gene expression profiling. Gastroenterology 2013;145(6):1289–99.
90. Furuta GT, Kagalwalla AF, Lee JJ, et al. The oesophageal string test: a novel, minimally invasive method measures mucosal inflammation in eosinophilic oesophagitis. Gut 2013;62(10):1395–405.
91. Katzka DA, Geno DM, Ravi A, et al. Accuracy, safety, and tolerability of tissue collection by cytosponge vs endoscopy for evaluation of eosinophilic esophagitis. Clin Gastroenterol Hepatol 2015;13(1):77–83.e2.
92. Bochner BS, Gleich GJ. What targeting eosinophils has taught us about their role in diseases. J Allergy Clin Immunol 2010;126(1):16–25 [quiz: 26–7].
93. Stein ML, Collins MH, Villanueva JM, et al. Anti-IL-5 (mepolizumab) therapy for eosinophilic esophagitis. J Allergy Clin Immunol 2006;118(6):1312–9.
94. Straumann A, Conus S, Grzonka P, et al. Anti-interleukin-5 antibody treatment (mepolizumab) in active eosinophilic oesophagitis: a randomised, placebo-controlled, double-blind trial. Gut 2010;59(1):21–30.
95. Assa'ad AH, Gupta SK, Collins MH, et al. An antibody against IL-5 reduces numbers of esophageal intraepithelial eosinophils in children with eosinophilic esophagitis. Gastroenterology 2011;141(5):1593–604.
96. Spergel JM, Rothenberg ME, Collins MH, et al. Reslizumab in children and adolescents with eosinophilic esophagitis: results of a double-blind, randomized, placebo-controlled trial. J Allergy Clin Immunol 2012;129(2):456–63, 463.e1-3.
97. Blanchard C, Mingler MK, Vicario M, et al. IL-13 involvement in eosinophilic esophagitis: transcriptome analysis and reversibility with glucocorticoids. J Allergy Clin Immunol 2007;120(6):1292–300.
98. Rothenberg ME, Wen T, Greenberg A, et al. Intravenous anti-IL-13 mAb QAX576 for the treatment of eosinophilic esophagitis. J Allergy Clin Immunol 2015; 135(2):500–7.
99. Mitson-Salazar A, Yin Y, Wansley DL, et al. Hematopoietic prostaglandin D synthase defines a proeosinophilic pathogenic effector human T(H)2 cell subpopulation with enhanced function. J Allergy Clin Immunol 2016;137(3):907–18.e9.
100. Straumann A, Hoesli S, Bussmann C, et al. Anti-eosinophil activity and clinical efficacy of the CRTH2 antagonist OC000459 in eosinophilic esophagitis. Allergy 2013;68(3):375–85.
101. Otani IM, Nadeau KC. Biologic therapies for immunoglobulin E-mediated food allergy and eosinophilic esophagitis. Immunol Allergy Clin North Am 2017; 37(2):369–96.
102. Al-Hussaini A, Al-Idressi E, Al-Zahrani M. The role of allergy evaluation in children with eosinophilic esophagitis. J Gastroenterol 2013;48(11):1205–12.
103. Wolf WA, Jerath MR, Sperry SL, et al. Dietary elimination therapy is an effective option for adults with eosinophilic esophagitis. Clin Gastroenterol Hepatol 2014; 12(8):1272–9.
104. van Rhijn BD, Vlieg-Boerstra BJ, Versteeg SA, et al. Evaluation of allergen-microarray-guided dietary intervention as treatment of eosinophilic esophagitis. J Allergy Clin Immunol 2015;136(4):1095–7.e3.
105. Kagalwalla AF, Amsden K, Shah A, et al. Cow's milk elimination: a novel dietary approach to treat eosinophilic esophagitis. J Pediatr Gastroenterol Nutr 2012; 55(6):711–6.

Food Protein-Induced Enterocolitis Syndrome

Theresa A. Bingemann, MD[a,b], Puja Sood, MD[b], Kirsi M. Järvinen, MD, PhD[b,*]

KEYWORDS

- Non-IgE–mediated food allergy
- Food protein-induced enterocolitis syndrome (FPIES) • Cow's milk • Soy
- Oral food challenge • Failure to thrive

KEY POINTS

- Awareness of food protein-induced enterocolitis syndrome is low.
- Food protein-induced enterocolitis syndrome (FPIES) can present as a medical emergency with symptoms including delayed persistent emesis with or without bloody diarrhea that can lead to severe dehydration and hemodynamic instability with abnormal laboratory markers.
- The mainstay of management is trigger avoidance.
- The natural history of the disease is spontaneous resolution over time.
- More studies are needed to better drive evidence-based practices for FPIES in clinical practice.

INTRODUCTION

Food protein-induced enterocolitis syndrome (FPIES) was first formally recognized by Powell in the 1970s.[1] FPIES is a non-immunoglobulin E (IgE)–mediated food allergy characterized by repetitive vomiting and frequent diarrhea that may lead to dehydration, lethargy, and pallor in the acute form. The chronic form is characterized by failure to thrive, emesis, and diarrhea. An atypical form, in which there is concomitant presence of specific IgE to the triggering food, has also been described.[2] Limited prevalence data exist, but this disorder is thought to be relatively rare.[3] The diagnosis is often missed likely because of the broad differential, delayed presentations, and limited awareness in the medical community.[4,5] Furthermore, the diagnosis is based solely on clinical criteria because no confirmatory test exists.[6] Implicated foods, onset

Disclosures: None.
[a] Allergy, Immunology and Rheumatology, Rochester Regional Health, 222 Alexander Street, Suite 3000, Rochester, NY 14607, USA; [b] Division of Pediatric Allergy and Immunology, University of Rochester School of Medicine and Dentistry, Rochester, NY 14642, USA
* Corresponding author. University of Rochester School of Medicine and Dentistry, 601 Elmwood Avenue, Box 611, Rochester, NY 14642.
E-mail address: Kirsi_jarvinen-seppo@URMC.Rochester.edu

Immunol Allergy Clin N Am 38 (2018) 141–152
https://doi.org/10.1016/j.iac.2017.09.009
0889-8561/18/© 2017 Elsevier Inc. All rights reserved.

of the disorder, and time to resolution vary by geographic area and regional dietary practices.[2,3,7,8] Treatment consists of education and avoidance of the offending foods. Many questions remain regarding this syndrome, and further research is needed.

EPIDEMIOLOGY

Food allergy prevalence has overall been increasing over the last 10 to 20 years.[9] FPIES, a non-IgE–mediated food allergy, has been reported as rare, although more than 1000 cases have been reported and cases reported per year have varied from 1 to 90.[10] There are few studies reviewing the prevalence of FPIES, and the true prevalence is unknown. The single population-based birth cohort study to date is by Katz and colleagues[3] in Israel, who prospectively studied 13,019 infants for development of FPIES related to cow's milk over 2 years. The study results showed a cumulative incidence for FPIES of 0.34% (44/13,019), with 8 of these patients subsequently developing IgE-mediated cow's milk allergy. In comparison, 0.5% (66/13,019) of the study population had IgE-mediated cow's milk protein allergy. All patients were diagnosed within the first 6 months of life in the study; however, the age of presentation can vary anywhere from 7 days of life to about 12 months of age.[2,3,8] Multiple studies report a male predominance similar to IgE-mediated food allergy.[3,8,11] There is an increased incidence of comorbid atopic disease in infants with FPIES, with about 30% of infants having atopic dermatitis, asthma, allergic rhinitis, or IgE-mediated food allergy.[8,11,12] Family history of atopy is common (40%–80%) in infants with FPIES; however, there are no cases of parents of infants with FPIES having had childhood or adult-onset FPIES, suggesting a lack of familial association.[10,12]

DIAGNOSIS
Symptoms

FPIES usually presents between 2 and 7 months of age as formulas and solid foods are introduced into the infant's diet. Milk and soy protein are the most common causes, although several studies also report reactions to other foods, including rice, oat, or other cereal grains, such as barley and wheat.[3,11,13] Children may have multiple food triggers. Cow's milk and soy FPIES often present at an earlier age than solid food-induced FPIES to grains, which is likely due to earlier introduction of cow's milk and soy. There are geographic variations of food triggers and age of diagnosis, likely based on differences in dietary implementation practices, with solid food-induced FPIES being more common in Europe and Australia than in North America (**Table 1**).[14] FPIES can present with both acute and chronic symptoms that are reflective of the non-IgE–mediated process and usually lack the typical expected IgE-mediated symptoms.

Acute symptoms

FPIES usually presents initially in infancy as severe emesis with or without diarrhea that may contain blood or mucous with exposure to the causative food (**Table 2**). The severe emesis is repetitive and may include up to 15 to 20 episodes of projectile repetitive vomiting within 1 to 4 hours of ingesting the suspected food.[4,9,14] The timing of onset of symptoms is important for the diagnosis. Secondary to these symptoms, children may have pallor, lethargy, metabolic acidosis, and hypothermia.[8,9,14] Laboratory abnormalities also include an increased neutrophil count, which peaks at 6 hours, and thrombocytosis (>500 × 10^9/L).[8] Often with this presentation, infants will undergo evaluation for sepsis, especially if marked laboratory abnormalities and hemodynamic

Table 1
Geographic variance of *typical* cow's milk/soy-induced versus solid-food induced food protein-induced enterocolitis syndrome

References and Year	Country	Number of Patients	Foods Assessed	Age at Onset of Diagnosis (CM/Soy)	Age at Onset of Diagnosis (Solid Food)
Sicherer et al,[2] 1998	United States	n = 16	Cow's milk, soy, solid foods	Median = 6 wk Mean = 7.52 wk	Median = 22 wk Mean = 22 wk
Nowak-Wegrzyn et al,[7] 2003	United States	n = 14	Solid foods	—	Median = 22 wk Mean = 20.6 wk
Fogg et al,[16] 2006	United States	n = 19	Cow's milk, soy, solid foods	Median = 8 wk Mean = 8.1 wk	Median = 18 wk Mean = 22.5 wk
Ruffner et al,[19] 2013	United States	n = 462	Cow's milk, soy, solid foods	Mean = 28 wk	Mean = 48.4 wk
Caubet et al,[11] 2014	United States	n = 160	Cow's milk, soy, solid foods	Mean = 20 wk	Mean = 28 wk
Mehr et al,[8] 2009	Australia	n = 35	Cow's milk, soy, solid foods	Median = 16 wk Mean = 19.6 wk	Median = 23.6 wk Mean = 24.4 wk
Hwang et al,[13] 2009	South Korea	n = 23	Cow's milk, soy	Mean = 5.14 wk	—
Katz et al,[3] 2011	Israel	n = 44	Cow's milk	Median = 4.3 wk Mean = 8.3 wk	—
Sopo et al,[20] 2012	Italy	n = 66	Cow's milk vs other foods	Mean = 14 wk (CM only)	Mean = 42.4 wk

Table 2
Symptoms of food protein-induced enterocolitis syndrome

Acute FPIES	Chronic FPIES
Vomiting in the 1- to 4-h period after ingestion of the suspected food	• Intermittent emesis
± Diarrhea within 24 h, usually 5–10 h, occasionally bloody	• Progressive diarrhea, ± blood
Decreased activity level/lethargy	• Lethargy/fatigue
Pallor	• Dehydration
Dehydration/hypovolemic shock with hypotension	• Poor growth/failure to thrive
Hypothermia	
Laboratory findings • Increased neutrophil count of ≥1500 neutrophils above baseline • Thrombocytosis • Metabolic acidosis • Methemoglobinemia • Stool + for leukocytes, eosinophils, or increased carbohydrate content	Laboratory findings • Thrombocytosis • Metabolic acidosis • Methemoglobinemia • Hypoalbuminemia

Adapted from NIAID-Sponsored Expert Panel, Boyce JA, Assa'ad A, et al. Guidelines for the diagnosis and management of food allergy in the United States: report of the NIAID-sponsored expert panel. J Allergy Clin Immunol 2010;126(6 Suppl):S1-58; with permission.

instability are present.[2] Diarrhea may be delayed and may occur 5 to 10 hours after ingestion of trigger foods. There is often no report of abnormal longitudinal growth or failure to thrive.[14]

Chronic symptoms
Chronic FPIES can vary in its clinical presentation and is not as well defined as acute FPIES (see **Table 2**). Chronic FPIES usually presents in neonates (less than 4 months of age) who were fed with cow's milk–based or soy-based formula from a young age.[4] These patients usually develop a more progressive diarrhea with intermittent emesis over time.[14] Poor weight gain and failure to thrive are common. However, patients can still present with ill appearance early in life, including lethargy, dehydration, metabolic acidosis, and methemoglobinemia.[4,9,14] They can also have laboratory aberrancies such as anemia, hypoalbuminemia, and an elevated white blood count with left shift and eosinophilia.[4] Despite their ill appearance, neonates or infants with chronic FPIES will improve once the offending food or foods are eliminated from the diet.

Diagnostic Criteria
International consensus guidelines outline that the diagnosis can often be made based on clinical history and noted improvement in symptoms once the suspected trigger or triggers have been removed from the diet, with an oral food challenge (OFC) as the gold standard for the confirmation of the diagnosis if there is uncertainty (**Table 3**). Given the relative rarity of the syndrome and lack of laboratory diagnostic tools for FPIES, it can be difficult to diagnose FPIES and can often be a diagnosis of exclusion. History taking should include a complete narrative of all possible reactions with a detailed record of symptoms, timing of symptoms in relation to food intake, a list of notably suspicious possible food triggers, and an indication of a pattern of reactions related to a specific food or foods.[15] It is in very rare cases that invasive procedures

Table 3
Diagnostic criteria of food protein-induced enterocolitis syndrome

Reproducible Reactions to Suspected Foods Based on History or Oral Food Challenge	
Acute FPIES	**Chronic FPIES**
Major criteria: Vomiting in the 1- to 4-h period after ingestion of the suspected food without typical IgE-mediated skin or respiratory symptoms Minor criteria: 1. Episode(s) of repetitive vomiting after eating the same suspected food 2. Repetitive vomiting episode 1 to 4 h after eating a different food 3. Presentation of lethargy with any suspected reaction 4. Presentation of pallor with any suspected reaction 5. Presentation requiring an emergency room visit with any suspected reaction 6. Presentation requiring fluid resuscitation with any suspected reaction 7. Diarrhea presenting within 24 h of ingestion of suspected food (usually 5–10 h) 8. Hypotension 9. Hypothermia 10. Increased neutrophil count of ≥1500 neutrophils above the baseline count The diagnosis of FPIES requires that a patient meets the major criterion and ≥3 minor criteria	• Intermittent but progressive vomiting and diarrhea (± blood) • Poor weight gain/failure to thrive • Dehydration • Metabolic acidosis • Resolution of symptoms within days after elimination of the offending food or foods and with recurrence of symptoms upon reintroduction • Requires confirmatory challenge

Adapted from NIAID-Sponsored Expert Panel, Boyce JA, Assa'ad A, et al. Guidelines for the diagnosis and management of food allergy in the United States: report of the NIAID-sponsored expert panel. J Allergy Clin Immunol 2010;126(6 Suppl):S1-58; with permission.

such gastrointestinal endoscopy is required.[6] If performed, friable mucosa, rectal ulceration, and bleeding can be seen with biopsies showing villous atrophy, tissue edema, crypt abscesses, and increased inflammatory cells.[4] There are no specific imaging studies for FPIES. It is important to continue to follow up with the patient at regular intervals and consider reintroduction or OFC to the causative food or foods to see if the allergy has resolved.[6] Although skin prick testing and specific IgE testing are negative in this non-IgE–mediated food allergy, it may be helpful to obtain skin prick testing in infants and children with comorbid conditions, such as atopic dermatitis or other signs of atopy. Children with FPIES may have detectable levels of specific IgE to the triggering food at presentation or on follow-up assessment; in this case the patient is defined as having "atypical FPIES."[15]

Atopy patch testing has been evaluated for its ability to predict reactivity to a food in FPIES at baseline,[16] with no value in predicting tolerance development in follow-up,[16,17] but data are scarce and the test is not in clinical use. The International Consensus Guidelines recommend an OFC to confirm the diagnosis if the causative food is unclear, if the symptom time course is unusual, or if there is lack of symptom resolution with removal of the suspected food from the diet. For many years the Powell criteria were used to define a positive challenge (3 or more of the following): vomiting, diarrhea, fecal blood (visible or occult), fecal leukocytes, fecal eosinophils, and a significant increase in the polymorphonuclear cell count greater than 3500 cells/mm^3.[18] The International Guidelines present revised diagnostic criteria to help interpret OFCs for patients with confirmed or possible FPIES (see **Table 3**). Major criterion for acute FPIES includes emesis within 1 to 4 hours after consumption of the food of concern without IgE-mediated respiratory or skin findings. Minor criteria include lethargy, pallor, diarrhea within 5 to 10 hours, low blood pressure, low body temperature, and an increase of ≥1500 neutrophils above the prechallenge count. If the major criterion and ≥2 of the minor criterion are met, the challenge is diagnostic of FPIES. Consideration must be given to therapies that may limit some of the signs and symptoms, like the use of ondansetron, and clinical judgment is needed in these circumstances. Outside of the research setting and in some centers, neutrophil counts may not be able to be performed promptly or the physician may choose not to not to pursue this.

For chronic FPIES, symptom resolution should occur within a few days of elimination of the food or foods of concern. If the suspected food is reintroduced to the diet, acute vomiting occurs within 1 to 4 hours after ingestion and diarrhea within 24 hours (more commonly between 5 and 10 hours, as above). The investigators point out the heterogeneity in presentation from milder forms, with intermittent emesis and/or diarrhea and typically poor weight gain, to severe forms, which also include metabolic acidosis, dehydration, and possibly bloody diarrhea.[9]

DIFFERENTIAL DIAGNOSIS

The differential diagnosis of FPIES is broad, encompassing multiple gastrointestinal, metabolic, allergic, infectious, cardiovascular, and neurologic disorders.[4] Fiocchi and colleagues[5] explored the diagnosis most often offered in acute and chronic presentations of FPIES in the literature. In the acute form, in order of decreasing frequency, the diagnosis offered was sepsis, acute gastroenteritis with dehydration, necrotizing enterocolitis, pyloric stenosis, intussusception, allergic proctocolitis, anaphylaxis, volvulus, epilepsy, food poisoning, Munchausen syndrome, and neurologic causes of shock. In the chronic form, the diagnosis offered was eosinophilic esophagitis, eosinophilic enterocolitis, eosinophilic gastroenteritis, celiac disease, gastroesophageal reflux, food allergy, metabolic disorders, food intolerances, primary immunodeficiency, and alpha-1 antitrypsin deficiency.

FOOD TRIGGERS

The most common causal food internationally is cow's milk.[8,11,19,20] Soy is the next most common causal food in the United States, but is not as common in other countries, where the most common foods vary relative to feeding practices and exposure. In Australia, rice was reported as the most common food trigger followed by soy and cow's milk.[8] In the United States, the next most common foods after milk and soy are grains such as rice and oat, which are typically the first weaning foods, followed by eggs, meats/fish, vegetables, fruits, peanuts, and tree nuts.[11,19] In Italy, fish was the second most common food reported.[20] FPIES to fish,[21] shellfish,[21,22] and mollusks has been described in adults.[21,23]

Internationally, patients vary in the number of trigger foods. The retrospective study of 35 children with FPIES in Australia, 83% reacted to a single food and the remainder had reactions to 2 foods.[8] In Italy, the retrospective study by Sopo and colleagues[20] found that 15% reacted to more than one food. In contrast, 2 studies in the United States showed a higher percentage of patients with FPIES reacting to more than one food. Caubet and colleagues[11] found in a retrospective study of 160 subjects, that most patients (65%) reacted to one food, 26% reacted to 2 foods, and 9% had reactions to 3 or more foods. Diagnosis was based on OFC (30%) or typical symptoms following ingestions within the preceding 12 months (70%). In another retrospective US study of 462 patients, 70% of subjects reacted to 1 or 2 foods, and approximately 30% reacted to 3 or more individual foods as determined by reproducible history of prolonged vomiting that may or may not have been accompanied by diarrhea 2 to 6 hours after ingesting the implicated food.[19]

ACUTE MANAGEMENT

When a patient experiences an acute reaction, traditionally intravenous (IV) fluids (10–20 mL/kg boluses of normal saline) have been recommended. Oral rehydration can be considered for mild reactions.[3] IV corticosteroid medications (methylprednisolone 1 mg/kg, up to 60–80 mg) have been recommended for more severe reactions. Chronic FPIES with dehydration and the most severe acute reactions may require vasopressors for hypotension not responsive to fluids, bicarbonate for academia, and methylene blue for methemoglobinemia. Recently, the use of ondansetron has been tried as well. Hollbrook and colleagues[24] report resolution of symptoms in an acute FPIES reaction during an OFC within 15 minutes of the administration of IV ondansetron in 5 children aged 3 to 12 years. They suggest the use of ondansetron for accidental ingestions and during OFCs. Subsequently, Miceli Sopo and colleagues[25] reported resolution of symptoms within 15 minutes with intramuscular (IM) ondansetron in 5 patients aged 12 months to 4 years. A retrospective, nonrandomized study of 66 children comparing the use of IV or IM ondansetron with traditional treatment showed a relative risk reduction of 0.2 favoring the ondansetron group, when comparing vomiting after the administration of therapy.[26] Of note, treatment was not successful in all cases, and they were unable to predict efficacy by timing of administration or patient factors. Leonard and Nowak-Wegrzyn[27] reports empiric use of oral ondansetron in at home reactions and cautions that medical evaluation should be sought as well.

DIETARY MANAGEMENT AND TREATMENT

Strict avoidance of the offending foods in all forms is the first line of treatment in managing FPIES. Some investigators have reported tolerance of the triggering food in baked goods in a few patients; however, this has not been found with all patients.[28] Furthermore, others have reported reacting to lower doses of the trigger food with subsequent exposures.[29–31] In acute and chronic FPIES to cow's milk, a hypoallergenic formula is often used because U.S. studies have shown that 40% to 50% of these patients will react to soy as well.[7,11,19] Studies from Israel,[3] Australia,[8] and Italy[20] have not found the same association between cow's milk and soy FPIES. In a population-based study designed to explore the prevalence and natural history of FPIES to cow's milk discussed earlier, no patient reacted to soy or other foods.[3] The difference in reactivity may be a result of differences in genetics, feeding practices, exposure patterns, or patient selection/referral patterns.[4] As such, one could consider soy as a cow's milk substitute if an OFC is performed (at home or in a supervised setting at the discretion of a physician) without an incident. An extensively hydrolyzed casein formula can be used as well.[2,7] Approximately 20% of infants with cow's milk FPIES will not tolerate this and will need an amino acid formula.[15,32,33]

It has been recognized that patients with cow's milk FPIES are also at greater risk of solid food FPIES. This number was higher with concomitant atopic dermatitis.[33]

One-third of infants with cow's milk or soy FPIES developed FPIES to a solid food.[33] In more recent series, the rate of reaction to a solid food in milk and soy FPIES was about 25%.[11] In the study by Sicherer,[33] 32% of children with liquid FPIES also developed solid food FPIES. Interestingly, in another study, many of the patients with solid food FPIES were already found to be on an extensively hydrolyzed formula and reacted to a median of 4 (range 1–5) solid food proteins.[7] However, although about one-third of children with cow's milk FPIES may react to solids, patients with solid food FPIES may not have as frequent reactions to liquids. A recent retrospective chart review of 39 patients diagnosed with FPIES found that most patients with oat FPIES tolerated cow's milk.[34] Ultimately, larger, multicenter studies will be needed to clarify the rate of multisensitization in FPIES using standard criteria.

The goal of dietary management is to avoid acute and chronic reactions, while using the least restrictive diet. For patients with early-onset FPIES, breastfeeding or an extensively hydrolyzed formula is recommended for this group in the first year of life.[15,33] A small percentage of patients will require an amino acid formula.[15,32,33] The consensus guidelines for FPIES suggest introducing complementary foods, when a child is developmentally ready at around 6 months of age. Consideration can be given to starting with lower-risk fruits and vegetables, followed by meats and cereals with each new food introduced over a period of 4 days.[15,35] Tolerating one food from a group is thought to convey a favorable prognosis for the other foods in the group. To promote healthy dietary variety and unnecessary limitation, super-vised challenges to one or mixed foods can be considered for patients that had severe cow's milk or soy FPIES. Accordingly, the International Guidelines[15] for a 1-year-old with FPIES suggest considering a challenge to high-risk foods not already introduced, singly or together, depending on the level of concern for a reaction. Because children frequently have to avoid several food items or groups, consideration should be given to dietician involvement to make sure nutritional needs are met.[36]

Breastfeeding is generally thought to be protective with respect to FPIES in that it is rare to see this entity in breastfed babies.[7,12] A few cases of FPIES due to cow's milk or soy have been described while breastfeeding.[29,30,37] In the very rare cases when patients experience a classic FPIES reaction when exposed to the allergic trigger pro-tein in breast milk, maternal restriction is recommended. Although studies are lacking on the best approach, many practitioners would allow maternal consumption of the trigger food if this has been tolerated.[4,29]

OFCs are used to confirm the diagnosis, assess for tolerance of foods within the same food group, and assess for resolution of FPIES.[27,36] Timing of challenge has not been systematically examined, and physician discretion, the impact of food avoid-ance, as well as family preference should also play a role in the decision of when to proceed with a challenge.[14] Sicherer[33] recommends considering a food challenge 12 to 18 months after the previous symptomatic ingestion in a facility with the ability to rapidly replace fluid loss. Significant dehydration due to recurrent emesis is seen in approximately half of reactive challenges,[4] and hypotension is seen in about 15%.[11] For FPIES, consideration should be given to placing an IV line before the chal-lenge given the risk for dehydration and hypotension especially if they have experi-enced previous severe reactions or might have difficult IV access.[15] After careful discussion with the family regarding the risk of a reaction, need of IV access, distance from care, previous reaction severity, and the trigger food, some practitioners may elect to allow home introduction.[15] Many protocols exist for performing OFCs for FPIES in the literature. Historically, 0.6 g of protein per kilogram of body weight was used to calculate dosing. Subsequently, it was recommended to use 0.15 to 0.3 g of protein per kilogram of body weight or less if the child has had a severe reaction or reacted with ingestion of a small amount of the food protein.[2,7,33] The doses are calculated based on the protein content of the food, and they recommend that the protein content of the challenge dose does not exceed 3 g protein or total food weight of 10 g. Three equal doses are administered over 30 to 45 minutes, and the patient is observed for 4 to 6 hours.[2,7,33,38]

Overall, it is difficult to predict the severity of a reaction. In one study, rice FPIES was associated with more severe reactions than milk and soy.[8,39] Nowak-Wegrzyn and colleagues[7] compared patients with milk or soy FPIES with patients with solid food FPIES and found a trend toward more severe reactions in solid food FPIES; however, this was not statistically significant ($P = .2$).[7] Most of the 462 patients in the study by Ruffner and colleagues[19] had a relatively mild phenotype, and only 5% presented with pallor, hypotension, or cyanosis.[19] In the study by Katz and colleagues,[3] 44 patients were diagnosed with milk FPIES, and details of physician-supervised OFCs were provided for 24 symptomatic patients all of whom were successfully treated with oral rehydration, suggesting milder presentation.

NATURAL HISTORY

Time to resolution of FPIES varies according to the food, area of the world, the presence of IgE, atopic dermatitis, methodological/protocol differences, referral patterns, and type of center the data comes from.[4,8,33] Time to resolution for cow's milk FPIES has ranged from 10 months in 90% of the patients in Korea to 3 years in 90% of patients in Israel, and to 5 years in 85% of patients in the United States {3, 13, 19, }. For soy, the earliest age resolution was similarly seen in Korea with resolution at 10 months of age in 90% of patients and the latest age of resolution in a US tertiary referral center at 6 to 7 years{13,11}. The early rate of resolution of cow's milk and soy FPIES in Korea may be explained by the earlier age at performance of food challenges. They were performing OFCs 6 months after their diagnosis and every 2 months after that, which is more frequent than practices reported elsewhere.[13]

Regarding solid food FPIES, resolution of rice FPIES occurred by 3 years in 80% in the study by Mehr[8] from Australia but only in 40% in the study by Caubet and colleagues[11] from the United States. In the United States, resolution for vegetables and oat occurs by 3 years in two-thirds of patients.[7] However, in a subsequent US report, resolution in grain FPIES was seen only by 5 years in two-thirds of the patients. In this report, an average age to tolerance with oat was 4 years and rice 4.7 years.[19] Jarvinen and Nowak-Wegzyn[4] caution that for foods that were easy to avoid and not considered essential to the diet, challenges were often deferred perhaps making age of resolution appear later. Meat FPIES resolved in 50% of patients in 5 years, but no cases of fish FPIES resolved in that same time period in the U.S. study.

Those patients with concomitant IgE sensitization (ie, "atypical" FPIES) remained symptomatic to the trigger food until a later age.[2] Of patients with persistent milk FPIES at age 3 years, 46% had detectable IgE to milk, whereas those who experienced resolution did not.[11] Conversely, one-fourth of FPIES patients had a positive food-specific IgE, mostly milk or soy, and one-third of these patients progressed to immediate symptoms with milk. Onesimo and colleagues[40] described children with cow's milk FPIES and specific IgE to milk who developed IgE-mediated symptoms on subsequent exposure. As a result, it is prudent to check specific IgE before challenge, particularly to milk. If IgE is detectable, the challenge should be modified to follow suggested protocols for an IgE-mediated allergy and treatment of anaphylaxis should be available.

SUMMARY AND FUTURE CONSIDERATIONS

Dietary education and avoidance of the trigger foods are the first-line treatment. Assessment with respect to growth is prudent. Consultation with a dietician to further assess nutritional adequacy can be helpful if the child is avoiding multiple foods or common ingredients.[36,41] Direction on emergency management should be provided to patients including a letter describing the syndrome and treatment to the emergency personnel.[15,33] As addressed previously, fluid resuscitation, corticosteroid medications, and possibly ondansetron can be used in FPIES. Unless a patient has atypical FPIES with the presence of specific IgE, epinephrine and antihistamines typically do not have a role in FPIES management.

The diagnosis of FPIES is based on clinical criteria. In the future, validation of these clinical criteria is needed. Ideally, a diagnostic test would be developed to help with the diagnosis,[15,42] and further studies addressing the pathophysiology of this syndrome are needed.[42] The optimum frequency and protocols for OFCs need to be determined.[15,42] More epidemiologic studies are needed to help with the prevalence, risk factors, natural history, and the impact of the disease.[39,42] Further studies are also needed on how strict dietary avoidance needs to be such as whether baked foods need to be avoided and in which patients. Until then, a high clinical suspicion is needed not to miss the diagnosis of FPIES, and a thoughtful approach to OFCs and follow-up is needed to avoid unnecessary food avoidance.

REFERENCES

1. Powell GK. Enterocolitis in low-birth-weight infants associated with milk and soy protein intolerance. J Pediatr 1976;88(5):840–4.
2. Sicherer SH, Eigenmann PA, Sampson HA. Clinical features of food protein-induced enterocolitis syndrome. J Pediatr 1998;133(2):214–9.
3. Katz Y, Goldberg MR, Rajuan N, et al. The prevalence and natural course of food protein-induced enterocolitis syndrome to cow's milk: a large-scale, prospective population-based study. J Allergy Clin Immunol 2011;127(3):647–53.e1-3.
4. Jarvinen KM, Nowak-Wegrzyn A. Food protein-induced enterocolitis syndrome (FPIES): current management strategies and review of the literature. J Allergy Clin Immunol Pract 2013;1(4):317–22.
5. Fiocchi A, Claps A, Dahdah L, et al. Differential diagnosis of food protein-induced enterocolitis syndrome. Curr Opin Allergy Clin Immunol 2014;14(3):246–54.
6. Sampson HA, Aceves S, Bock SA, et al. Food allergy: a practice parameter update-2014. J Allergy Clin Immunol 2014;134(5):1016–25.e43.
7. Nowak-Wegrzyn A, Sampson HA, Wood RA, et al. Food protein-induced enterocolitis syndrome caused by solid food proteins. Pediatrics 2003;111(4 Pt 1): 829–35.
8. Mehr S, Kakakios A, Frith K, et al. Food protein-induced enterocolitis syndrome: 16-year experience. Pediatrics 2009;123(3):e459–64.
9. NIAID Sponsored Expert Panel, Boyce JA, Assa'ad A, et al. Guidelines for the diagnosis and management of food allergy in the United States: report of the NIAID-sponsored expert panel. J Allergy Clin Immunol 2010;126(6 Suppl):S1–58.
10. Mehr S, Frith K, Campbell DE. Epidemiology of food protein-induced enterocolitis syndrome. Curr Opin Allergy Clin Immunol 2014;14(3):208–16.
11. Caubet JC, Ford LS, Sickles L, et al. Clinical features and resolution of food protein-induced enterocolitis syndrome: 10-year experience. J Allergy Clin Immunol 2014;134(2):382–9.

12. Nowak-Wegrzyn A, Muraro A. Food protein-induced enterocolitis syndrome. Curr Opin Allergy Clin Immunol 2009;9(4):371–7.
13. Hwang JB, Sohn SM, Kim AS. Prospective follow-up oral food challenge in food protein-induced enterocolitis syndrome. Arch Dis Child 2009;94(6):425–8.
14. Nowak-Wegrzyn A, Jarocka-Cyrta E, Moschione Castro A. Food protein-induced enterocolitis syndrome. J Investig Allergol Clin Immunol 2017;27(1):1–18.
15. Nowak-Wegrzyn A, Chehade M, Groetch ME, et al. International consensus guidelines for the diagnosis and management of food protein-induced enterocolitis syndrome: executive summary–Workgroup Report of the Adverse Reactions to Foods Committee, American Academy of Allergy, Asthma & Immunology. J Allergy Clin Immunol 2017;139(4):1111–26.e4.
16. Fogg MI, Brown-Whitehorn TA, Pawlowski NA, et al. Atopy patch test for the diagnosis of food protein-induced enterocolitis syndrome. Pediatr Allergy Immunol 2006;17(5):351–5.
17. Jarvinen KM, Caubet JC, Sickles L, et al. Poor utility of atopy patch test in predicting tolerance development in food protein-induced enterocolitis syndrome. Ann Allergy Asthma Immunol 2012;109(3):221–2.
18. Powell GK. Food protein-induced enterocolitis of infancy: differential diagnosis and management. Compr Ther 1986;12(2):28–37.
19. Ruffner MA, Ruymann K, Barni S, et al. Food protein-induced enterocolitis syndrome: insights from review of a large referral population. J Allergy Clin Immunol Pract 2013;1(4):343–9.
20. Sopo SM, Giorgio V, Dello Iacono I, et al. A multicentre retrospective study of 66 Italian children with food protein-induced enterocolitis syndrome: different management for different phenotypes. Clin Exp Allergy 2012;42(8):1257–65.
21. Tan JA, Smith WB. Non-IgE-mediated gastrointestinal food hypersensitivity syndrome in adults. J Allergy Clin Immunol Pract 2014;2(3):355–7.e1.
22. Gleich GJ, Sebastian K, Firszt R, et al. Shrimp allergy: gastrointestinal symptoms commonly occur in the absence of IgE sensitization. J Allergy Clin Immunol Pract 2016;4(2):316–8.
23. Fernandes BN, Boyle RJ, Gore C, et al. Food protein-induced enterocolitis syndrome can occur in adults. J Allergy Clin Immunol 2012;130(5):1199–200.
24. Holbrook T, Keet CA, Frischmeyer-Guerrerio PA, et al. Use of ondansetron for food protein-induced enterocolitis syndrome. J Allergy Clin Immunol 2013; 132(5):1219–20.
25. Miceli Sopo S, Battista A, Greco M, et al. Ondansetron for food protein-induced enterocolitis syndrome. Int Arch Allergy Immunol 2014;164(2):137–9.
26. Miceli Sopo S, Bersani G, Monaco S, et al. Ondansetron in acute food protein-induced enterocolitis syndrome, a retrospective case-control study. Allergy 2017;72(4):545–51.
27. Leonard SA, Nowak-Wegrzyn A. Food protein-induced enterocolitis syndrome. Pediatr Clin North Am 2015;62(6):1463–77.
28. Miceli Sopo S, Buonsenso D, Monaco S, et al. Food protein-induced enterocolitis syndrome (FPIES) and well cooked foods: a working hypothesis. Allergol Immunopathol (Madr) 2013;41(5):346–8.
29. Tan J, Campbell D, Mehr S. Food protein-induced enterocolitis syndrome in an exclusively breast-fed infant-an uncommon entity. J Allergy Clin Immunol 2012; 129(3):873 [author reply: 873–4].
30. Monti G, Castagno E, Liguori SA, et al. Food protein-induced enterocolitis syndrome by cow's milk proteins passed through breast milk. J Allergy Clin Immunol 2011;127(3):679–80.

31. Bansal AS, Bhaskaran S, Bansal RA. Four infants presenting with severe vomiting in solid food protein-induced enterocolitis syndrome: a case series. J Med Case Rep 2012;6:160.
32. Vanderhoof JA, Murray ND, Kaufman SS, et al. Intolerance to protein hydrolysate infant formulas: an underrecognized cause of gastrointestinal symptoms in infants. J Pediatr 1997;131(5):741–4.
33. Sicherer SH. Food protein-induced enterocolitis syndrome: case presentations and management lessons. J Allergy Clin Immunol 2005;115(1):149–56.
34. Kapoor M, Bird JA. Cow's milk protein is often tolerated by children with oat-induced FPIES. J Allergy Clin Immunol Pract 2017;5(2):496–7.
35. Groetch M, Henry M, Feuling MB, et al. Guidance for the nutrition management of gastrointestinal allergy in pediatrics. J Allergy Clin Immunol Pract 2013;1(4): 323–31.
36. Boyce JA, Assa'ad A, Burks AW, et al. Guidelines for the diagnosis and management of food allergy in the United States: summary of the NIAID-sponsored expert panel report. J Allergy Clin Immunol 2010;126(6):1105–18.
37. Kaya A, Toyran M, Civelek E, et al. Food protein-induced enterocolitis syndrome in two exclusively breastfed infants. Pediatr Allergy Immunol 2016;27(7):749–50.
38. Nowak-Wegrzyn A, Assa'ad AH, Bahna SL, et al. Work Group report: oral food challenge testing. J Allergy Clin Immunol 2009;123(6 Suppl):S365–83.
39. Mehr SS, Kakakios AM, Kemp AS. Rice: a common and severe cause of food protein-induced enterocolitis syndrome. Arch Dis Child 2009;94(3):220–3.
40. Onesimo R, Dello Iacono I, Giorgio V, et al. Can food protein induced enterocolitis syndrome shift to immediate gastrointestinal hypersensitivity? A report of two cases. Eur Ann Allergy Clin Immunol 2011;43(2):61–3.
41. Venter C, Groetch M. Nutritional management of food protein-induced enterocolitis syndrome. Curr Opin Allergy Clin Immunol 2014;14(3):255–62.
42. Wang J, Fiocchi A. Unmet needs in food protein-induced enterocolitis syndrome. Curr Opin Allergy Clin Immunol 2014;14(3):206–7.

Unproven Diagnostic Tests for Food Allergy

Catherine Hammond, MD, Jay A. Lieberman, MD*

KEYWORDS

- Food allergy • Diagnosis • Atopy patch test • IgG testing • Provocation
- Electrodermal • Cytotoxic • Kinesiology

KEY POINTS

- Atopy patch testing for food allergies is debatable, and may have an adjunct role in atopic dermatitis and eosinophilic esophagitis.
- Skin prick testing, serum immunoglobulin E (IgE) testing, and oral food challenges remain the currently accepted tests for immediate (anaphylactic) type food allergies.
- Serum IgG testing, provocation/neutralization, electrodermal testing, cytotoxic testing, and applied kinesiology are unproven and currently unaccepted methods to diagnose food allergy.

INTRODUCTION

Although the self-reported prevalence of food allergy is as high as 10% in Westernized countries such as the United States, the prevalence of actual diagnosed food allergy is lower.[1] This discordance often drives patients (and parents of patients) with suspected food allergy to pursue a variety of diagnostic procedures in search of answers and advice. Currently, the gold standard for the diagnosis of food allergy is the oral food challenge (OFC), whereas serum immunoglobulin E (IgE) and skin prick testing (SPT) serve as accepted readily available markers of sensitization to help predict clinical reactivity and obviate challenges. Unfortunately, serum and SPT are only useful for the diagnosis and management of IgE-mediated food allergies, and they have little or no role in diagnosing other food hypersensitivity disorders or intolerances, and the oral challenge can be time consuming, fear inducing, and possibly not readily available to many patients. Thus, many patients may seek alternative diagnostic methods for their (or their child's) suspected food allergy. In fact, based on one report, nearly 1 in 5 patients with self-reported food allergy has undergone unproven

Disclosures: Dr J.A. Lieberman and Dr C. Hammond have no disclosures or conflicts of interest related to this article or this publication.
Department of Pediatrics, The University of Tennessee Health Science Center, 51 North Dunlap, Suite 400, Memphis, TN 38105, USA
* Corresponding author.
E-mail address: Jlieber1@uthsc.edu

diagnostic testing.[2] This testing, if not proven, clearly has the possibility of leading to incorrect diagnoses, unnecessary elimination diets, and altering the quality of life for patients and families. Therefore, it is critical for providers (and arguably patients) to understand the methodology and research behind both proven and unproven techniques in order to counsel patients appropriately. This article briefly reviews proven techniques of food allergy testing for IgE-mediated allergies and focuses on debatable or unproven techniques.

PROVEN TECHNIQUES FOR TESTING IMMUNOGLOBULIN E–MEDIATED FOOD ALLERGY

The following testing modalities are recommended in current guidelines and practice parameters of various organizations and countries and are universally accepted by expert consensus panels on the diagnosis of food allergy (specifically IgE-mediated food allergy).[3–5]

Skin Prick Testing

A positive SPT response indicates the presence of IgE specific to the antigen in question and represents an observable physiologic response to that allergen. Although SPTs for foods have high sensitivity, they have low specificity and should therefore be correlated with the patient's history to determine clinical relevance.[6]

Food-Specific Serum Immunoglobulin E

Food-specific serum IgE (sIgE) testing is also accepted as an appropriate first-line test for food allergy and is often used in conjunction with SPT. Similarly to SPT, it also has low specificity and should be interpreted in light of the patient's history.

As an aside, it is worth mentioning that sIgE panels to a large number of foods appear to be increasingly popular, especially among primary care providers.[7] Panel testing has led to an increased cost per patient, overdiagnosis of food allergy, and unnecessary elimination diets in addition to an emotional and financial burden for patients and their families.[8] Although these tests are widely available and easy to perform, the use of food allergen sIgE panels is discouraged.

Oral Food Challenges

The double-blind, placebo-controlled food challenge (DBPCFB) is widely accepted as the gold standard for diagnosis food allergy, and there are available reports and guidelines to aid clinicians in performing these appropriately.[9,10] However, DBPCFB is both labor and time intensive, so the open OFC is more often used in the clinical setting; however, one must be aware that the open OFC can be affected by both patient and observer bias.

OTHER FOOD ALLERGY DIAGNOSTIC MODALITIES

Many of the diagnostic techniques discussed in this section either have not been studied in rigorous trials or have conflicting data regarding their utility.

Patch Testing

Atopy patch testing (APT) is a diagnostic procedure for delayed hypersensitivity reactions and is commonly used in the diagnosis of contact dermatitis. It has been studied in various forms of food allergy, but it must be noted that the methods and interpretation of results have yet to be standardized for foods and APT may be especially difficult to interpret in patients with underlying atopic dermatitis (AD), where irritant reactions could be interpreted as false positive results. In addition, given that APT is directed at a specific hypersensitivity reaction, the utility of the test for food allergy will greatly depend on the population studied and what type of "food allergy" for which the patients are undergoing testing.

"Mixed" allergy

Some researchers have examined the utility of APT as a diagnostic marker for food allergy with varying clinical presentation. For example, Caglayan-Sozmen and colleagues[11] examined the diagnostic utility of APT and SPT in comparison with OFC in children with suspected egg or milk allergy with varying clinical presentations (including eczema, urticaria, anaphylaxis, proctocolitis, and so forth). The results showed that APT had a low sensitivity, specificity, positive predictive value (PPV), and negative predictive value (NPV) for both milk and egg, and, thus, the investigators concluded that there was insufficient evidence to support the use of APT in predicting the outcome of OFC to these foods. Another study of children with varying presentations of suspected food allergy to milk, egg, wheat, or soy also showed that APT alone was of little diagnostic utility.[12] When examining these studies, however, one must realize that by enrolling children with varying clinical presentations, some may have had IgE-mediated disease and some cell-mediated diseases; thus, the ability of APT to perform for a specific condition is difficult to interpret from these studies.

Although the above studies suggest that APT was not useful in evaluating patient groups with a wide range of presentations, it may be more useful in patients with more specific complaints suspected to be secondary to a non-IgE–mediated reaction to foods. For example, in one study of diagnostic tests in patients with food-related gastrointestinal symptoms (excluding eosinophilic esophagitis [EoE]), the combination of SPT/APT was shown to have a high sensitivity and NPV.[13] Another study also found the SPT/APT combination had a high sensitivity; however, this study found that the combination had a low NPV, and thus it did not decrease the need for OFC in these patients.[14]

Patch testing has also been studied in food protein-induced enterocolitis syndrome (FPIES), another non-IgE–mediated food hypersensitivity. FPIES presents a diagnostic dilemma because there is no useful diagnostic tool short of an OFC, which carries risk of severe reactions, with up to half of patients requiring fluid resuscitation after a positive challenge.[15] One study found that APT had high NPV (100%) and PPV (75%) and thus could be a helpful tool in determining the need for OFC.[16] However, a similar study found that APT had NPV of only 55% and PPV 40%, perhaps because of different methods of interpreting APT results between the 2 studies.[15] Clearly, more research needs to be done in the non-IgE–mediated food hypersensitivity patient population (and a better understanding of the pathophysiology of the disease being tested is needed) before a clear recommendation can be made.

Atopic dermatitis

Patients with AD represent a particularly interesting subset of food allergy patients, given that their manifestations can represent an overlap of IgE-mediated and cell-mediated reactions to foods.[17] Therefore, one could reason that these patients warrant food allergy testing beyond SPT and/or sIgE in order to optimize treatment. Various studies have examined the use of APT in subjects with AD and suggest that it may be helpful in this patient population as an adjunct test along with sIgE or SPT.[18–22]

One of the earlier studies done on food APT in patients with AD evaluated children 2 to 36 months of age with both SPT and APT for milk before an OFC. Although SPT could predict acute-onset reactions, APT was often positive (89%) in subjects with delayed-onset reaction (worsening of AD). The investigators concluded that using both SPT and APT together can enhance the accuracy of diagnosis of milk allergy in AD patients.[18] A similarly designed study evaluating SPT and APT for milk, egg, wheat, and soy also found that using both tests together was helpful in predicting a positive OFC. Furthermore, these investigators suggested that using APT as a predictor for positive delayed-onset OFC may help prevent unnecessary elimination diets based on history alone.[19] More recently, one group compared APT and SPT when examining AD flares over time. The results suggested that APT and SPT performed nearly identically when examining all tests/foods, and the investigators also suggested that when both tests are positive, all patients had a positive OFC.[22] Similar results have been found in studies that combine APT with sIgE testing, suggesting that APT plus sIgE can help predict AD flares due to foods and may help obviate OFC.[20,21]

As always, there are limitations to the previously mentioned studies. First, they were all done in pediatric AD patients. Second, there is yet to be a standardized protocol for completing and interpreting APT for foods. Third, one must be able to tease out when the studies are specifically looking at the utility of the test for AD flares (delayed reactions), or if they examine the utility of APT in immediate reactions as well, as the pathophysiology of these are quite different.

Eosinophilic esophagitis

APT is also beginning to gain popularity in management of food elimination in patients with EoE. It has been shown that elimination diets are successful in producing histologic remission of EoE, seen in approximately 90% of those on elemental diet and 70% of those on 6-food elimination diet (SFED).[23] Clearly, a test-based, guided diet would be ideal; however, to date, there is no single best test to determine this. In the most recent consensus guidelines for EoE in fact, there is no recommendation on how to test for food allergies in EoE or how to use these tests for dietary modifications.[24]

Most of the reports on APT in patients with EoE have come from a single center.[25–28] The most recent retrospective report from that center analyzed 941 patients with EoE. All patients underwent SPT and APT to a panel of foods (unless already positive based on SPT). The investigators identified a cohort of 319 patients in whom causative foods had been identified based on diet and biopsy and used this population to calculate NPV and PPV of the SPT, APT, and the combination of the 2. In contrast to AD studies wherein the combination led to a high PPV, the investigators found that the SPT/APT combination in EoE had a high NPV (greater than 96% for all foods tested except milk, egg, and wheat) but a low PPV (42% or lower, with the exception of milk at 82% and egg at 61%). More importantly, they concluded that elimination diets based on SPT/APT results were equally successful (based on histology) as the SFED but accomplished this with elimination of a fewer number of foods.[28] One other institution reporting results of SPT/APT-driven diets in a retrospective study also suggested that a diet based on removal of foods that were positive on SPT and/or APT led to similar remission rates as compared with the SFED.[29] A third group has shown that the use of a combination of SPT/APT to guide elimination diet in children with EoE can lead to an improvement in symptoms, regardless of disease severity, and allowed for a reduction or discontinuation of pharmacotherapy.[30]

The utility of APT in EoE may be limited to a pediatric population, however. In one study of SPT/APT in an adult population with EoE, none of the subjects had a positive APT to the foods in the SFED. Those with positive SPT had similar success with SPT-driven elimination diet as those in the SFED group, and the SPT-driven diet group achieved these results with elimination of a fewer number of foods.[31]

Conclusions on patch testing

The current literature clearly has conflicting evidence on the utility of APT in the diagnosis of food allergy. Furthermore, there are no standardized food reagents for APT and significant variability in APT interpretation. Therefore, there is insufficient evidence to suggest that it, especially when used alone, is a useful tool in the diagnosis of food allergy. Although it may have some limited utility in predicting delayed positive reaction to OFC in the setting of AD and/or EoE, future research remains to be done.

Food-Specific Serum Immunoglobulin G

Several studies have demonstrated that production of food-specific IgG is the body's natural response to a regularly ingested food,[32–37] and recent studies have shown that IgG to cow's milk protein can be detected in 98% of healthy children by 2 years of age.[37] In addition, there are no established, standardized reference values for IgG specific for foods.[38] Despite these facts, large panel assays are readily available to providers. Most laboratories and clinicians that offer these tests suggest that they are not meant to diagnose immediate, anaphylactic-type food allergies, but rather that they can be used to diagnose other, chronic-food mediated disease, for example, irritable bowel syndrome (IBS), chronic fatigue, migraines, and so forth. Although studies examining the utility of food-specific IgG testing in these various conditions do exist, there are no well-designed trials using DBPCFC, and many of the studies are not controlled studies. Thus, the results must be taken cautiously.

Irritable bowel syndrome

It is clear that symptoms of IBS can be related to food, and dietary therapy for IBS is a treatment option.[39] In addition, many patients with IBS strongly believe that food intolerance contributes to their symptoms and report improvement with elimination diets.[40] Thus, although allergists are not typically trained to diagnose and manage IBS, many patients may seek the care of allergists for diagnosis and management if they think that "food allergies" are causing their symptoms.

Some researchers have postulated that IBS symptoms may be mediated by IgG antibodies and thus could be immune mediated. For example, in perhaps the most widely cited of these articles, Atkinson and colleagues[41] enrolled 150 patients with IBS into a randomized controlled trial of elimination diet based on elevated IgG values or to a sham diet. The subjects who eliminated foods to which they had elevated IgG values had a 10% reduction in symptom score when compared with subjects who consumed a sham diet. In a similar study of patients with both IBS and migraines, IgG-based elimination diet also led to subjective improvement in both disorders.[42] These findings, however, if accurate and reproducible, do not mean that IgG antibodies are pathogenic in IBS and offer no data to suggest a true hypersensitivity or immune response to the foods in question.

Other suspected allergic conditions

In addition to IBS, other chronic conditions have been studied in relation to food-specific IgG. Dixon[43] reported results of IgG-based food elimination diet in 114 patients who were suspected of having a "delayed food allergy" based on any of a wide variety of reported symptoms, such as gastrointestinal discomfort, nasal congestion, headaches, chronic fatigue, and behavioral problems. Participants underwent IgG testing to 10 to 15 foods that they consumed at least twice weekly and subsequently were instructed to eliminate foods that the author considered to have significantly elevated IgG levels. Eighty patients reported dietary compliance for a minimum of 4 months, and 71% of these patients were considered to have a successful outcome (defined as a 75% improvement in original symptoms). This study has been cited as evidence that IgG testing may be helpful in evaluation of suspected food allergy. There are several limitations to this study that cannot be overlooked, however. First, there was no control group (sham diet or other). Thus, there was likely a very high placebo effect in these patients with subjective symptoms alone. Second, there was no reintroduction or challenge to prove symptoms returned on ingestion. Third, there were no biomarkers checked prediet or postdiet to detect any objective effect. Fourth, there was no strict protocol for these patients, and this was not a prospective study; rather it was a single author's experience and reportedly did not require institutional board review. Thus, when examining these data, it is clear that further, more rigorous studies are needed in this area if any positive conclusions can be drawn.

Immunoglobulin E–mediated allergy

To date, there are no data linking food-specific IgG to immediate-type reactions. In fact, on the contrary, allergen-specific IgG4 is commonly accepted as a marker of tolerance induced by allergen immunotherapy, and many recent studies on food allergy immunotherapy (whether by oral, epicutaneous, or sublingual route) support this concept.[44–48]

Interestingly, one side effect of food allergy immunotherapy (at least oral immunotherapy) has been EoE.[49] Although the pathogenesis is not fully understood, there are now various studies suggesting that IgG4 to foods may actually play a role in the pathogenesis and/or the symptomatology of EoE.[50,51] Clearly, more data are needed in this regard, but it does perhaps provide one small framework in which IgG may be a useful marker in at least one form of food allergy.

Conclusions on serum food specific immunoglobulin G

Based on available data, there clearly is no role for IgG testing for immediate-type food reactions. For delayed "food allergies" or chronic complaints that may be related to foods, there are some studies that have suggested that dietary modification based on IgG testing does lead to symptom improvement; however, one must realize that these studies are likely to be biased because of the placebo effect, and more rigorous studies are clearly needed to support its use.

Provocation and Neutralization

Provocation tests are conducted by exposing a patient to an antigen (sublingually or intradermal) and observing for 10 minutes. Any symptom (dry mouth, headache, anxiety, and so forth) reported by the patient during this observation period is interpreted as a positive test. The provocation test is sometimes followed by a neutralization procedure during which the same antigen is given in a different dose until the reaction is "neutralized."[52,53] Test doses are not standardized and often are not used with a negative control. Two randomized, double-blind, placebo-controlled studies showed that a similar percentage of patients reacted to the antigen as they did to placebo.[54,55] Based on these results, it is reasonable to conclude that provocation/neutralization should not be used as a form of detection/intervention. Furthermore, the use of neutralization can potentially lead to severe adverse reaction in those patients with true IgE-mediated food allergy, with one case showing that it was associated with a near-fatal reaction in a patient who had unrecognized symptoms that were eventually diagnosed as systemic mastocytosis.[56]

Pulse Testing

Sometimes used as an additional objective measure during provocation-neutralization testing, the pulse test is considered positive if the heart rate changes 16 beats per minute after a sublingual or intradermal dose of food (or also during OFC). As best the authors can tell, the test interestingly has its roots in a book written by Dr Arthur Coca in 1956.[57] However, outside of this book, which is not a report of research (rather a description of a technique he used in various patients with various complaints), the authors can find no research articles actually examining this technique. Thus, there is no standardized technique, and there are no blinded studies examining its reliability or validity. Although this test seems to still be a popular technique in alternative/complementary medicine, there is little scientific evidence to support its use.

Electrodermal Testing

Electrodermal testing (ET) is performed by measuring skin conductance in an electrical circuit that contains an aluminum plate in contact with a sealed vial of food extract; a drop in conduction (presumably indicating disruption to the electric field) is interpreted as an allergy.[58] Perhaps the earliest scientific analysis of this method reported the ability to discriminate allergic versus nonallergic subjects up to 96% of the time using a double-blind study method.[59] However, since that study, other studies have suggested otherwise. One double-blind, placebo-controlled study on ET to diagnose respiratory allergy showed that the method not only has poor reproducibility but also that it could not reliably differentiate between allergens and negative controls.[60] Another double-blind, randomized study concluded that ET was unable to differentiate atopic and nonatopic patients.[61] Although it has not been studied specifically for food allergy, the available literature shows that ET is neither valid nor accurate.

Cytotoxic Testing

Cytotoxic testing is based on the hypothesis that when exposed to a noxious substance (in this case, a suspected allergen), leukocyte morphology changes. Initially, microscopy was used to detect these morphologic changes. One study in 1976, using a control population as well as a food-allergic group, concluded that there was no correlation between test results and clinical picture; furthermore, there was a high rate of false positives and inconsistency in interpreting results (even among tests read multiple times by the same investigator).[62] Another controlled double-blinded study also found no correlation between test results and clinical symptoms.[63] More recently, studies were done using flow cytometry to assess morphologic changes in cells after exposure to food antigen and have also found this method to be inconclusive and controversial.[64,65]

Despite the above, the antigen leukocyte antibody test (ALCAT), a commercial blood test that uses flow cytometry and cell impedance technology, remains easily obtainable by patients and claims to diagnose food sensitivity, with some panels testing more than 200 foods.[66] Based on an individual's sensitivity results, a diet is designed. The company acknowledges that their product does not test for IgE-mediated food allergy, but does not release information regarding the methodology or reliability/validity of their test. Furthermore, the literature provided by the company to support its use, including reports using double-blind studies, could not be accessed in PubMed or have only been presented in abstract form and have not been published as a peer-reviewed journal article.

Applied Kinesiology Testing

Applied kinesiology (AK) testing is performed by having a patient hold a vial containing an allergen in question while the muscle strength in the opposite arm is measured (by the test performer applying a light pressure to that arm); a positive test is indicated by a decrease in strength of the tested arm.[67] Several studies regarding the utility of this form of testing have been published by the International College of Applied

Kinesiology; however, a review of the literature published in this field during the 1980s showed that the vast majority of these studies were based on poor research designs and/or poor reporting techniques.[68] One recent blinded study done to assess the test-retest reliability and validity of kinesiology testing in the diagnosis of venom allergy concluded that "kinesiology as a diagnostic tool is not more useful than random guessing."[69] Similarly, another double-blind randomized study to assess the validity of AK testing also concluded that it was an unreliable tool.[70] Little research has been done on the usefulness of AK testing in the diagnosis of food allergy.

FUTURE CONSIDERATIONS/SUMMARY

The most current expert consensus panels agree that although the DBPCFC remains the gold standard for food allergy diagnosis, sIgE and SPT are acceptable alternatives.[3,4] Although largely considered unreliable, the other previously discussed unproven methods of food allergy testing are still available and are often appealing to patients. Although APT, and possibly food-specific IgG testing, may be of some benefit when used in conjunction with other proven methods in certain patient populations, more research needs to be done in this area. Experts agree that APT may have limited utility in guiding dietary management of pediatric EoE, but it is still not recommended for routine use in food allergy diagnosis.[4] The other techniques discussed have largely been discredited or are unproven and are not recommended.

REFERENCES

1. Savage J, Johns CB. Food allergy: epidemiology and natural history. Immunol Allergy Clin North Am 2015;35:45–59.
2. Ko J, Lee JI, Munos-Furlong A, et al. Use of complementary and alternative medicine by food-allergic patients. Ann Allergy Asthma Immunol 2006;97:365–9.
3. Boyce JA, Assa'ad A, Burks AW, et al. Guidelines for the diagnosis and management of food allergy in the United States: report of the NIAID-sponsored expert panel. J Allergy Clin Immunol 2010;126(Suppl 6):S1–58.
4. Sampson HA, Aceves S, Bock SA, et al. Food allergy: a practice parameter update-2014. J Allergy Clin Immunol 2014;134:1016–25.
5. Muraro A, Werfel T, Hoffmann-Sommergruber K, et al. EAACI food allergy and anaphylaxis guidelines: diagnosis and management of food allergy. Allergy 2014;69:1008–25.
6. Weiser KS, Takwoingi YT, Panesar SS, et al. The diagnosis of food allergy: a systematic review and meta-analysis. Allergy 2014;69:76–86.
7. Stukus DR, Kempe E, Leber A, et al. Use of food allergy panels by pediatric care providers compared with allergists. Pediatrics 2016;138(6) [pii:e20161602].
8. Bird JA, Crain M, Varshney P. Food allergen panel testing often results in misdiagnosis of food allergy. J Pediatr 2015;166:97–100.
9. Nowak-Wegrzyn A, Assa'ad AH, Bahna SL, et al. Work Group report: oral food challenge testing. J Allergy Clin Immunol 2009;123(6 Suppl):S365–83.
10. Sampson HA, Gerth van Wijk R, Bindslev-Jensen C, et al. Standardizing double-blind, placebo-controlled oral food challenges: American Academy of Allergy, Asthma & Immunology-European Academy of Allergy and Clinical Immunology PRACTALL consensus report. J Allergy Clin Immunol 2012;130:1260–74.
11. Caglayan-Sozmen SC, Dascola CP, Gioia E, et al. Diagnostic accuracy of patch test in children with food allergy. Pediatr Allergy Immunol 2015;26:416–22.

12. Mehl A, Rolinck-Werninghaus C, Staden U, et al. The atopy patch test in the diagnostic workup of suspected food-related symptoms in children. J Allergy Clin Immunol 2006;118:923–9.
13. Canani RB, Ruotolo S, Auricchio L, et al. Diagnostic accuracy of the atopy patch test in children with food allergy-related gastrointestinal symptoms. Allergy 2007; 62:738–43.
14. Boonyaviwat O, Pacharn P, Jirapongsananuruk O, et al. Role of atopy patch test for diagnosis of food allergy-related gastrointestinal symptoms in children. Pediatr Allergy Immunol 2015;26:737–41.
15. Järvinen KM, Caubet JC, Sickles L, et al. Poor utility of atopy patch test in predicting tolerance development in food protein-induced enterocolitis syndrome. Ann Allergy Asthma Immunol 2012;109:221–2.
16. Fodd MI, Brown-Whitehorn TA, Pawlowski NA, et al. Atopy patch test for the diagnosis of food protein-induced enterocolitis syndrome. Pediatr Allergy Immunol 2006;17:351–5.
17. Tam JS. Cutaneous manifestation of food allergy. Immunol Allergy Clin N Am 2017;37:217–31.
18. Isolauri E, Turjanmaa K. Combined skin prick and patch testing enhances identification of food allergy in infants with atopic dermatitis. J Allergy Clin Immunol 1996;97:9–15.
19. Niggemann B, Reibel S, Wahn U. The atopy patch test (APT) – a useful tool for the diagnosis of food allergy in children with atopic dermatitis. Allergy 2000;55:281–5.
20. Roehr CC, Reibel S, Ziegert M, et al. Atopy patch tests, together with determination of specific IgE levels, reduce the need for oral food challenges in children with atopic dermatitis. J Allergy Clin Immunol 2001;207:548–53.
21. Chung BY, Kim HO, Park CW, et al. Diagnostic usefulness of the serum-specific IgE, the skin prick test and the atopy patch test compared with that of the oral food challenge test. Ann Dermatol 2010;22(4):404–11.
22. Visitsunthorn N, Chatpornvorarux S, Pacharn P, et al. Atopy patch test in children with atopic dermatitis. Ann Allergy Asthma Immunol 2016;117:668–73.
23. Arias A, González-Cervera J, Tenias JM, et al. Efficacy of dietary interventions for inducing histologic remission in patients with eosinophilic esophagitis: a systematic review and meta-analysis. Gastroenterology 2014;146(7):1639–48.
24. Liacouras CA, Furuta GT, Hirano I, et al. Eosinophilic esophagitis: updated consensus recommendations for children and adults. J Allergy Clin Immunol 2011;128(1):3–20.
25. Spergel JM, Beausoleil JL, Mascarenhas M, et al. The use of skin prick tests and patch tests to identify causative foods in eosinophilic esophagitis. J Allergy Clin Immunol 2002;109:363–8.
26. Spergel JM, Andrews T, Brown-Whitehorn TF, et al. Treatment of eosinophilic esophagitis with specific food elimination diet directed by a combination of skin prick and patch tests. Ann Allergy Asthma Immunol 2005;95:336–43.
27. Spergel JM, Brown-Whitehorn T, Beausoleil JL, et al. Predictive values for skin prick test and atopy patch test for eosinophilic esophagitis. J Allergy Clin Immunol 2007;119:509–11.
28. Spergel JM, Brown-Whitehorn TF, Cianferoni A, et al. Identification of causative foods in children with eosinophilic esophagitis treated with an elimination diet. J Allergy Clin Immunol 2012;130(2):461–7.
29. Henderson CJ, Abonia JP, King EC, et al. Comparative dietary therapy effectiveness in remission of pediatric eosinophilic esophagitis. J Allergy Clin Immunol 2012;129(6):1570–8.

30. Syrigou E, Angelakopoulou A, Zande M, et al. Allergy-test-driven elimination diet is useful in children with eosinophilic esophagitis, regardless of the severity of symptoms. Pediatr Allergy Immunol 2015;26:323–9.

31. Rodriguez-Sanchez J, Torrijos EG, Viedma BL, et al. Efficacy of IgE-targeted vs empiric six-food elimination diets for adult eosinophilic esophagitis. Allergy 2014;69:936–42.

32. Host A, Husby S, Gjesinb G, et al. Prospective estimation of IgE, IgG subclass and IgE antibodies to dietary proteins in infants with cow milk allergy. Allergy 1992;47:218–29.

33. Keller KM, Burgin-Wolff A, Lippold R, et al. The diagnostic significance of IgG cow's milk protein antibodies re-evaluated. Eur J Pediatr 1996;155:331–7.

34. Jenmalm MC, Bjorksten B. Exposure to cow's milk during the first 3 months of life is associated with increased levels of IgG subclass antibodies to beta-lactoglobulin to 8 years. J Allergy Clin Immunol 1998;102:671–8.

35. Kruszewski J, Raczka A, Kłos M, et al. High serum levels of allergen specific IgG-4 (asIgG-4) for common food allergens in healthy blood donors. Arch Immunol Ther Exp (Warsz) 1994;42(4):259–61.

36. Schwarz A, Panetta V, Cappella A, et al. IgG and IgG4 to 91 allergenic molecules in early childhood by route of exposure and current and future IgE sensitization: results from the Multicentre Allergy Study birth cohort. J Allergy Clin Immunol 2016;138:1426–33.

37. Siroux V, Lupinek C, Resch Y, et al. Specific IgE and IgG measured by the MeD-ALL allergen-chip depend on allergen and route of exposure: the EGEA study. J Allergy Clin Immunol 2017;139:643–54.

38. Martins TB, Bandhauer ME, Wilcock DM, et al. Specific immunoglobulin (Ig) G reference intervals for common food, insect, and mold allergens. Ann Clin Lab Sci 2016;46:635–8.

39. Chey WD. Food: the main course to wellness and illness in patients with irritable bowel syndrome. Am J Gastroenterol 2016;111:366–71.

40. Nanda R, James R, Smith H, et al. Food intolerance and the irritable bowel syndrome. Gut 1989;30:1099–104.

41. Atkinson W, Sheldon TA, Shaath N, et al. Food elimination based on IgG antibodies in irritable bowel syndrome: a randomized controlled trial. Gut 2004;53:1459–64.

42. Aydinlar EI, Dikmen PY, Tiftikci A, et al. IgG-based elimination diet in migraine plus irritable bowel syndrome. Headache 2012;53:514–25.

43. Dixon HS. Treatment of delayed food allergy based on specific immunoglobulin G RAST testing. Otolaryngol Head Neck Surg 2000;123:48–54.

44. Vickery BP, Pons L, Kulis M, et al. Individualized IgE-based dosing of egg oral immunotherapy and the development of tolerance. Ann Allergy Asthma Immunol 2010;105:444–50.

45. Burks AW, Jones SM, Wood RA, et al. Oral immunotherapy for treatment of egg allergy in children. N Engl J Med 2012;367:233–43.

46. Jones SM, Ponsz L, Roberts JL, et al. Clinical efficacy and immune regulation with peanut oral immunotherapy. J Allergy Clin Immunol 2009;124:292–300.

47. Jones SM, Sicherer SH, Burks AW, et al. Epicutaneous immunotherapy for the treatment of peanut allergy in children and young adults. J Allergy Clin Immunol 2017;139(4):1242–52.

48. Fleischer DM, Burks AW, Vickery BP, et al. Sublingual immunotherapy for peanut allergy: a randomized, double-blind, placebo-controlled multicenter trial. J Allergy Clin Immunol 2013;131:119–27.

49. Lucendo AJ, Arias A, Tenias JM. Relation between eosinophilic esophagitis and oral immunotherapy for food allergy: a systematic review with meta-analysis. Ann Allergy Asthma Immunol 2014;113:624–9.

50. Clayton F, Fang JC, Gleich GJ, et al. Eosinophilic esophagitis in adults is associated with IgG4 and not mediated by IgE. Gastroenterology 2014;147:602–9.

51. Wright BL, Kulis M, Guo R, et al. Food-specific IgG4 is associated with eosinophilic esophagitis. J Allergy Clin Immunol 2016;138:1190–2.e3.

52. King WP, Rubin WA, Fadal RG, et al. Provocation-neutralization: a two-part study. Part I. the intracutaneous provocative food test: a multi-center comparison study. Otolaryngol Head Neck Surg 1988;99:263–71.

53. King WP, Rubin WA, Fadal RG, et al. Provocation-neutralization: a two-part study. Part II. subcutaneous neutralization therapy: a multi-center study. Otolaryngol Head Neck Surg 1988;99:272–7.

54. Jewett DL, Phil D, Fein G, et al. A double-blind study of symptom provocation to determine food sensitivity. N Engl J Med 1990;323:429–33.

55. Fox RA, Sabo BMT, Williams TPW, et al. Intradermal testing for food and chemical sensitivities: a double-blind controlled study. J Allergy Clin Immunol 1999;103:907–11.

56. Teuber SS, Vogt PJ. An unproven technique with potentially fatal outcome: provocation/neutralization in a patient with systemic mastocytosis. Ann Allergy Asthma Immunol 1999;82:61–5.

57. Coca AF. The pulse test. New York: Lyle Stuart Publishers; 1956.

58. Lewith GT. Can we evaluate electrodermal testing? Complement Ther Med 2003; 11:115–7.

59. Krop J, Lewith GT, Gziut W, et al. A double blind, randomized, controlled investigation of electrodermal testing in the diagnosis of allergies. J Altern Complement Med 1997;3:241–8.

60. Semizzi M, Senna G, Rapacioli G, et al. A double-blind, placebo-controlled study on the diagnostic accuracy of an electrodermal test in allergic subjects. Clin Exp Allergy 2002;32:928–32.

61. Lewith GT, Kenyon JN, Broomfield J, et al. Is electrodermal testing as effective as skin prick tests for diagnosing allergies? A double blind, randomized block design study. Br Med J 2001;(322):131–4.

62. Lieberman P, Crawford L, Bjelland J, et al. Controlled study of the cytotoxic food test. JAMA 1976;231:728–30.

63. Benson TE, Arkins JA. Cytotoxic testing for food allergy: evaluation of reproducibility and correlation. J Allergy Clin Immunol 1976;58:471–6.

64. Bindslev-Jensen C, Poulsen LK. What do we at present know about the ALCAT test and what is lacking? Monogr Allergy 1996;32:228.

65. Potter PC, Mullineux J, Weinberg EEG, et al. The ALCAT test inappropriate in testing for food allergy in clinical practice. S Afr Med J 1992;81:384.

66. Available at: https://cellsciencesystems.com/providers/alcat-test. Accessed May 15, 2017.

67. Garrow JW. Kinesiology and food allergy. Br Med J (Clin Res Ed) 1988;296:1573–4.

68. Klinkoski B, Lebouf C. A review of the research papers published by the International College of Applied Kinesiology from 1981 to 1987. J Manipulative Physiol Ther 1990;13(4):190–4.

69. Ludtke R, Kunz B, Seeber N, et al. Test-retest reliability and validity of the kinesiology muscle test. Complement Ther Med 2001;9:141–5.

70. Schwartz SA, Utts J, Spottiswoode SJ, et al. A double-blind, randomized study to assess the validity of applied kinesiology (AK) as a diagnostic tool and as a nonlocal proximity effect. Explore (N Y) 2014;10(2):99–108.

Moving?

Make sure your subscription moves with you!

To notify us of your new address, find your **Clinics Account Number** (located on your mailing label above your name), and contact customer service at:

Email: journalscustomerservice-usa@elsevier.com

800-654-2452 (subscribers in the U.S. & Canada)
314-447-8871 (subscribers outside of the U.S. & Canada)

Fax number: 314-447-8029

Elsevier Health Sciences Division
Subscription Customer Service
3251 Riverport Lane
Maryland Heights, MO 63043

*To ensure uninterrupted delivery of your subscription, please notify us at least 4 weeks in advance of move.

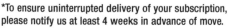